SAFE
AND
SOUND

Secrets of the World's Most Resilient People

Written by Russ Magnall

Safe & Sound

Secrets of the World's Most Resilient People

Second edition published in 2023

ISBN: 979-8-39291015-1

Imprint: Independently Published

ABOUT THE AUTHOR

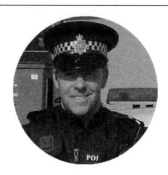

Russ Magnall is a former police commander with Greater Manchester Police. An unshakeable optimist who believes in a bright future and our ability to build it together.

Russ is experienced in emergency and neighbourhood policing and management of critical incidents as a joint emergency services commander. As a police dog handler for nine years, he perfected the search skills which took him through promotion and on to lead specialist counterterrorist search teams.

A founder member of the Greater Manchester Police Strategic Wellbeing board, he has significant experience delivering resilience training and is credited with the design and delivery of the **Bee Well** programme to support Greater Manchester Police officers and staff following the terrorist attack at the Manchester Arena in 2017.

Russ is a qualified organisational development coach, specialised in leadership and wellbeing and, having retired from the police after an exemplary thirty-year career, now delivers his unique Safe and Sound personal resilience training for organisations across the country.

Connect with Russ on LinkedIn: @RussMagnall

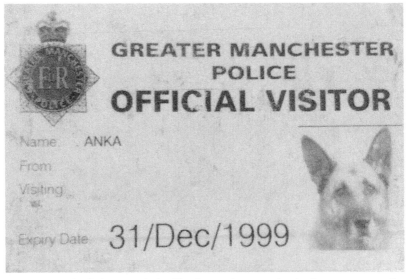

Identity card for Police dog Anka. The force photographer had a great sense of humour and thought Anka should have her own badge!

A NOTE ABOUT STRUCTURE

Despite my best efforts to structure this book in some sort of logical way it has, just like life, twisted, turned, stopped, started, and gone, at times, in completely different directions to what I first imagined!

What you can be sure of is that it will entertain you, make you smile, laugh and cry but, above all, show you how to cope well with day-to-day challenges and survive the biggest ones that test you to your limits. It is packed with stories, quotes, examples, tips, tools, and techniques all tested in the toughest arenas. It's the sort of book you can start from the front or the back or just pick up and read whichever page falls open! However you choose to read it, I know the content will help you live a happier, less stressful life. A life with meaning, purpose, and even more compassion for yourself and others. I hope you enjoy it.

CONTENTS

INTRODUCTION

The 10 December 1972 should have been an ordinary day. It wasn't. It was a day which turned my life upside down. The day started as a happy family day out in the beautiful North Yorkshire countryside and ended with the death of my mum in a head-on car crash on a narrow winding country road. I was eight years old. I was sitting in the back seat next to my younger sister. My stepdad was driving; my mum, in the passenger seat. I pause for a moment here to say that I'm not fishing for sympathy, far from it. I'm sharing a moment from my life which could have set me up for a life of misery, mayhem, and madness but didn't. Read on and I'll explain.

I have patchy memories of the hour that followed the crash, although it becomes crystal clear as I recall the events unfold the morning after. Waking up on a children's ward with my sister in the bed next to mine, I remember the sound of the crisp white curtain being drawn around the beds to shield us from the curious gaze of others as the doctor delivered his devastating news. During the nights which followed, I lay awake at night waiting for her spirit to come back to see me. She was bound to come back ... wasn't she?

I didn't know it then, but my mum's death would shape the person I would become. Fast forward to 1989 and the start of a thirty-year career as a Police Officer. That experience would help me to help others. I was able to connect with people and have difficult, compassionate conversations with people who had also lost loved ones in tragic circumstances, able to reassure them that in time their pain would ease, and they would be OK. I found I could find the right words to help them see the way forward. It was only after I'd retired from policing and was reflecting on my career that I realised just how much my mum's death had helped me to become a compassionate police officer, able to have those conversations, which in a strange, twisted way, was cathartic for me. It helped me because I was helping others.

My mum's death taught me that no matter how devastating the situation, there can be a way through. It taught me that sharing experience and talking about how you feel can heal. It taught me the value of positive communication, with myself and others, and how personal 'story' could be the greatest teacher. Most of all, it taught me never to give up hope. Hope was at the heart of everything I did as a police officer and remains at the heart of everything I do today.

It was a privilege to serve the communities of Greater Manchester. As a police commander I've led some of the finest men and women in the world, and I don't say that lightly. If you could spend just one day in their boots, you would understand. Men and women who have the same life challenges as you and me. Health issues, relationship stress, work and money worries, family problems, addictions, fears, and phobias as well as just about anything else you can think of! Men and women who also put on a uniform and go to work to face all manner of challenges and things too horrific to imagine. Did I mention that my team were one of the first to respond to the terrorist attack at the Manchester Arena on that fateful night of Monday, 22 May 2017?

My time in the police taught me how the most resilient police officers kept going no matter what life threw at them and filled my own resilience 'bank' with tips, tools, and techniques until it overflowed. It seems that the world could do with more resilience right now. Come with me and let me share what I know with you.

I'm going to share my journey with you. How I survived thirty years serving as a police officer on the streets of Manchester. How I coped with things too horrific to think about, a catalogue of catastrophic events in my personal life, and the day-to-day stuff which crops up for us all. I'll share what I saw and what I felt to help you avoid the pitfalls. I'll share what I learned working alongside some of the mentally strongest people I know. I'll share tips, tools, and techniques used by working in the toughest professions outside of policing, skills used by elite athletes as they prepare for the race of their life and fighter pilots taking fast jets to their limits. The same skills used by surgeons to steady their scalpel as they make that first incision and special forces soldiers as they focus on their mission.

Every one of the tips, tools, and techniques is scientifically proven and easy to learn. Skills I've used daily which you can use, immediately, to put you in the driving seat on the journey to improve your life, helping you build unshakeable personal resilience, strong mental health, and the ability to respond well to anything life throws at you.

Why?

Personal resilience is the ability to bounce back from adversity and leap forward to face life's challenges. It is the most important life skill. We need it to survive. Resilience is the golden thread weaving through every aspect of life. It helps us do well at school, choose the right friends and cope with peer pressure. It builds confidence, pushing us through exam stress and helps us develop strong, stable relationships which endure. Resilience decides how successful we are. It forges our character and reputation at home, at work, as a partner, parent, colleague, and friend. It galvanises our ability people al with whatever life throws at us from the day-to-day bumps in the road to catastrophic life-changing events. It helps us keep going. It is the critical life skill.

CHAPTER 1

Wellbeing

The better you cope, the better you feel. Personal resilience links directly to wellbeing and mental health and you don't have to look far to see the growing mental health crisis across the UK. Numerous studies evidence urgent need to improve wellbeing and mental health support for all, particularly young people who say that mental health is their number one concern and top of their agenda right now. The more resilient you are, the happier you will be.

Education

Personal resilience is rarely taught as a standalone subject. It's not part of the school curriculum yet has a massive impact on young lives. Students learn by trial and error, guided by teachers whose teaching time is dominated by academic priorities, targets and managing oversized classes. Resilience as a subject should be afforded greater recognition and dedicated space within the curriculum because of the impact it has on life. If we value our young people as much as we say we do, we should be listening to them. They are asking for this, and lessons in resilience will add more value to a young person's life than lessons in any other subject.

Resilience at work

Work-related stress accounts for over half of all working days lost to ill health in Great Britain. Over 17 million working days were lost in 2022, significantly higher than pre-pandemic levels. The financial impact on organisations and the impact on employee wellbeing is huge. High levels of personal resilience are vital if workplace performance is to soar and stress, anxiety, and days lost through psychological sickness are to drop.

Resilience at home

Family break-ups are at an all-time high. The walls of divorce courts could tell hundreds of stories of broken relationships where resilience crashed leaving people unable to cope. Thousands of tiny irritating moments built up over time, left to fester and grow, corroding relationships, and ripping families apart. Small things becoming the big things which turn happy homes into places of hostility and anguish, wrecking lives, and shattering dreams.

Stress in the home is hardly surprising when you see how stressed we are at work. Perhaps we come home to a partner who's had a bad day and feels at the end of their tether, a potential for disaster.

The bickering starts, something we've done (or not done) is the flame which lights the blue touch paper. A petty argument heats up, things spiral out of control with both parties unable (or unwilling) to put the brakes on. A money worry gets thrown into the growl, some poorly chosen words, a mistake from yesterday or a gremlin from the past waiting to ambush. An explosive combination which can be terminal for any relationship if not resolved properly.

If we don't have the skills to deal with these things properly, they will come up repeatedly, causing more distress and damage every time they do. Resilience is about managing the emotions which come with all these challenges to help people make the right choices. Resilience helps you navigate a safe path to stop the small things becoming the big things which destroy relationships. Resilient emotional management is a vital skill if we want our relationships to last.

Suicide is painless – or is it?

A difficult subject to talk about: the decision to die greater than the decision to live. A national issue of concern for our country today. Hope and resilience had drained away for nearly 8,000 people in the UK in 2018. Men, women, and children who couldn't cope and believed death was their only way out. Three-quarters of those who died were men.

One of the most difficult parts of being a police officer was dealing with suicide. Life is precious and I always felt devastated for the person in front of me and the people left behind. Suicide is never painless, despite the words in the song. When times get tough, give yourself some time. Talk to someone. Read this book and follow my journey through these pages. I will change your perception and show you better options to help you out of the darkness. Read on, I promise you will be glad you did, and so will the people who love you.

Summary

Resilience matters. It is not my intention to paint a bleak picture, but it is my intention to be honest and lay out why it's important. It doesn't matter who you are, what job you have, how powerful you are, or how much money you have in the bank. Nobody is immune from the devastation stress and poor mental health can cause. Resilience is the number one life skill. The armour protecting us from harm and the lifeboat keeping us afloat when we're sinking. It helps us succeed at work and thrive in our personal lives. It gives us the courage to follow our dreams, to drive through adversity and deliver our best. It makes us tolerant, compassionate, and strong. Resilience is our guardian angel, a constant companion giving us the confidence to believe, skills to achieve and the motivation to cope with anything life throws at us, and it matters – a lot.

Objectives

1. **To reflect on what you already know**

2. **To improve the skills you already have**

3. **To learn new tips, tools, and techniques.**

I've written this book making it easy to digest all at once or in bite-sized pieces. An aide-memoire and a book you can pick up, read a page, and immediately benefit. The sort of book to change the way you think and nourish you immediately. A book you can also leave lying around at home or work to spark conversations about resilience, wellbeing, or mental health. Half the battle is getting people to talk about these topics. and my hope above all else is that this book encourages people to talk.

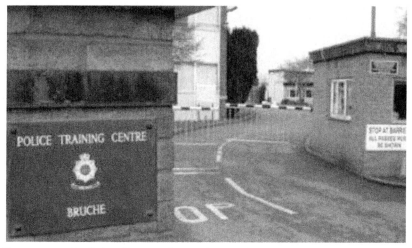

The gates to the Police Training Centre Bruche Warrington. Where it all started on 17th April 1989.

The railway story – things can only get better

It was my second day as an operational police officer and the ink was still wet on my warrant (identity) card. I was 'in company' with my tutor constable, an experienced police officer whose job it was to show me the ropes. We'd been on an early shift starting at 6 a.m. and were about to go home at 2 p.m. when the call came in: 'report of a deceased male on the railway line.'

There's something about 'jobs' like these. If there's a new probationer, or 'proby' as they were known, on duty when jobs like these came in, the new kid goes. Something about testing their mettle or some other rubbish reason for making you go to the most hideous incidents you can imagine! That day, the new kid was me. My tutor and I made our way to the railway line to be greeted by four hulking great railway workmen dressed in regulation British Rail kit. Steel toe cap boots, black work trousers, and donkey jackets covered by orange safety vests, all leaning on shovels and in good spirits thanks to this unplanned break in their day.

They nodded down the track towards a tunnel. It was a long tunnel. So long, in fact, that you couldn't see daylight at the other end. We began the long sombre walk along it, keeping between the steel tracks and pointing our heavy-duty torches in front of us so we didn't trip. It smelled damp and oily. I could hear water dripping off the roof and a cool breeze kissed my face as it drifted along the tunnel towards me. Our voices echoed as we talked nervously; it was eerie. The railway lads were following close behind. I was glad of their company. We were approaching a potential crime scene and, yes, it was highly likely that this person had taken their own life by jumping in front of the 13:35 to Manchester Victoria, but as a police officer, it had been drummed into me at training school to keep an open mind and let the facts tell the story. We went first. My tutor and I, side by side, approached the middle of the tunnel. It was pitch black.

My torch beam picked out the first clue to the horror about to unfold. A severed arm lying right in front of me across the metal line. I swallowed nervously. A bit further on and just to the right: a leg. And then the worst sight you can possibly imagine, a sight straight out of the scariest horror film you've ever seen. The battered torso of a fully grown man run over by a train. I felt like I was in some surreal nightmare; it didn't seem real. The torso looked like it had been slashed with a sword – a huge gaping wound running diagonally, shoulder to groin. The internal organs spilling out onto the ballast stones at the side of the tracks like the mangled mess of a butcher's display tossed into the air and left to splatter on the floor. His head was almost unrecognisable, squashed forward as if spread along the tracks by a huge knife as a knife spreads butter on bread.

The railway lads stood close by watching us work. Two of them eating sandwiches. I was being sick. I composed myself, and to this day I still don't know how. Up until that point, I'd only ever seen one dead body. Lying in repose in the chapel of rest. Neat, peaceful, and beautiful. My tutor guided me through the tried-and tested procedures for dealing with a sudden death in these circumstances. The Criminal Investigation Department detectives attended to ensure there was nothing suspicious or evidence of foul play; scenes of crime specialists, to gather evidence and take photographs; the undertaker, to remove the remains and transport in a body bag to the mortuary. The coroner's report was completed by us before retiring from duty.

As I left the station, my duty done for the day, my sergeant stopped me: 'All part of the job son. If you can't hack this sort of thing, you're in the wrong job. See you tomorrow!' And that was it! I paused a moment to let this uplifting, motivational, and compassionate piece of welfare advice sink in before walking out in a daze and getting in my car.

As I drove home, the images I saw in that tunnel played over and over in my mind. I wondered whether he jumped from the side or stood in the middle of the tracks? I thought about the train driver and wondered how he was. I wondered whether he heard the impact of the man hitting his train. I wondered if he saw the look on the man's face as he met his fate. It frightened me. I thought about the dead man's family. I imagined the devastation about to pour over them when one of my colleagues knocked on their door. I wondered how those workmen could eat their sandwiches.

It was probably a good two weeks before I slept properly after that. I was a sound sleeper normally, but every night the images exploded from my subconscious and into my nightmares. It was horrible but I got over it. Or did I?

In 1989, you were expected to keep a stiff upper lip and not to show your emotions, only talking about jobs like this in a macho, bravado kind of way, like nothing bothered you. And the welfare response back in those days?: 'Broad shoulders son, get yourself a beer. You'll be 'right.'

Today things are quite different. Officers and support staff experiencing any traumatic event can expect much better compassionate support. At the very least, a debrief at the end of the shift for you to talk about your experience, what happened, what you did, what you thought or felt, room. In fact, you can talk about anything you want. Talking is a good thing; it gives you chance to offload, to decompress. Decompress. I like that word. It's exactly the right word for this type of situation. I think we all need time and space to decompress occasionally, don't you?

What is personal resilience?

During my workshops, delegates are asked to consider five questions during the day. Each is delivered in a coaching style where they discuss with their colleagues and reflect on what personal resilience means to them. There are multiple right answers. The ability to cope. To be able to carry on. To not go sick. To let things 'go over your head'. You will have your own response to this question. My definition is this:

The ability to bounce back from life's challenges and bounce forward to face new ones.

The 'bounce forward' element is important. I want my officers to deal well and bounce back from life's challenges, but I also want them to be able to bounce forward to the next one. I want this for you too. I want you to try new things, to step out of your comfort zone, to go for that new job or promotion, to have the courage to embark on a new relationship, to bounce forward and try things which enhance and improve your story with unshakeable personal resilience giving you the confidence to go for it! The tips, tools, and techniques in here will help you do that.

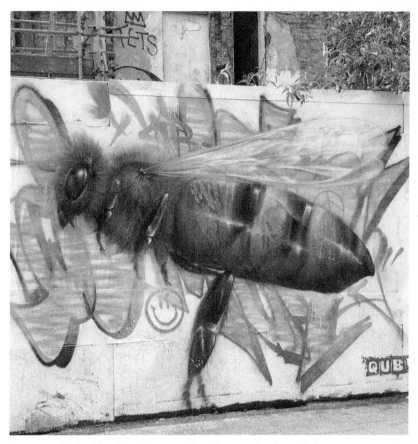

Street art in the Northern Quarter Manchester. The humble bee represents the industrial history of this great city and it's resilience following the terrorist attack at the Manchester Arena in 2017

Stress versus pressure

It's important to know the difference between stress and pressure because each has a quite different impact on your wellness.

Too much stress will grind you down and make you ill. Pressure is what makes stuff worth doing.

Pressure is a positive aspect of life and work for most people. Many of us need to have standards, targets, and deadlines to push us towards good performance. Pressure is what I feel as the need to perform – and everyone has an optimum level of pressure that brings about their best performance. It is pressure when I feel that it is achievable. I might have to work hard, take some risks, challenge myself, change or accept new things, but it is manageable – I feel I have control over the situation.

Stress, on the other hand, occurs when I no longer feel in control. That what is being demanded of me is not manageable, no matter how organised, effective, or efficient I become.

Distinguishing stress from pressure can prevent you becoming so worn out that you eventually burn out. The most important thing to remember is that no matter what stress hits you, there is a way of dealing with it.

Sometimes you don't realise the weight of something you've been carrying until you feel the weight of its release.

Day one

At any point on your journey through life, you can choose to change, step out of your comfort zone, and try a new approach. Reading this book may be your day one.

All new recruits receive self-defence training to help them deal with violent people. Unarmed tactics including wristlocks, blocks, arm entanglements (arm up the back technique if we're not being technical), breakaway techniques, and holds, swiftly moving on to handcuff techniques and how to use a truncheon! Trust me when I say it's not just as simple as hitting someone with it!

The police truncheon, like resilience and mental health support has evolved over the years. In 1989, to be honest, both were pretty useless. It's quite different today.

I've arrived at the public order training site in east Manchester, showed my warrant card and walked through the massive metal concertina doors into a huge warehouse where a variety of self-defence and public order drills take place.

It's a huge place. Imagine an aircraft hangar: concrete floor and walls with a high ceiling, probably a hundred feet above me. This hangar has twenty or so concrete rooms to replicate locations police officers might have to operate in. Cells, corridors, three-storey flats, terraced houses, and streets to practise protective shield work. I can hear instructors shouting in the distance, their booming voices echoing around the arena, and I'm feeling intimidated already.

I spot two instructors, well, more like two replica Incredible Hulks, sitting in a small wooden office to my right. Everything about this place looks rough, including these two.

'Excuse me mate, I'm here for my initial self-defence training; please can you tell me where to go?' I ask in as deep a voice as possible to try to give the impression I'm tougher than I am.

The reply immediately roars back at me.

'NUMBER ONE: I'M NOT YOUR MATE! … AND NUMBER TWO!' … (looking me up and down like I'm something from the gutter!) 'GET YOURSELF DOWN TO CLASSROOM NUMBER TWO – DOWN THERE ON THE LEFT IN TWO MINUTES LOOKING SOMETHING LIKE A POLICE OFFICER.'

'Seems friendly,' I think as I hurry to the classroom.

The day went well as we were taken through the basics. I've never been a 'fighting man' or considered myself a 'tough guy', so I was keen to learn from the experts, confident that what they taught me would keep me safe on the mean streets of Manchester.

The truncheon I'd been issued with was brand new, made of wood and lighter in weight than I'd imagined. Light brown in colour in contrast to the dark oak truncheons issued in the 1960s and 1970s which were a lot heavier and would have had far more clout. It mattered not. This was mine. The females were issued with an identical version except it was half the length to fit into their regulation issue handbags. Some of the boys found this funny. Most of the girls did not.

'RIGHT YOU LOT. GET YOUR STAFFS OUT,' (police terminology for truncheon) 'AND LINE UP' the instructor growled.

We did as we were told. Forty of us all fidgeting nervously with our brand-new staffs.

'I'M GOING TO SHOW YOU HOW TO DEFEND YOURSELF FROM ATTACK USING YOUR STAFF' he bawled.

He demonstrated how to wind the leather loop handle around your hand in such a way as to retain control of it with the strap should the aggressor grab it and try to take it off you whilst at the same time being able to disengage yourself from the staff and 'create space' if needed. This technique is sound and is still used to today with the modern-day metal extendable baton.

We were taught to hold the staff horizontally in front of us, a hand at either end.

'DEFENCE FROM A KICK TO THE GROIN!' he bellowed.

The low block. 'All together now'… 'LOW BLOCK,' we all shout out in unison.

And on this instruction, we all 'presented' our staffs in front of us, bending low as if to fend off an assailant aiming a kick at us. Brilliant! Have you ever seen this technique used on any of the reality police TV programmes on telly? No? There's a surprise!

'WELL DONE. YOU CAN, WITH MY BLESSING, APPLY FOR A PLACE ON MASTERMIND.'

He obviously considered us intelligent for being able to follow his instruction.

Medium block came next. Hold the staff in the same way but 'present' at waist height to repel a punch to the abdomen. Great stuff, and on his command: 'MEDIUM BLOCK'

Again, in perfect harmony, we all present our staffs. Seen this done for real on the telly? Probably not.

Final move of the three … yes, you've guessed it … the high block. Designed to defend against a knife attack from above. All together now… 'HIGH BLOCK' and once again we go top of the class for performing this choreographed move perfectly. Come on, you must have seen this one being done somewhere surely?

I had that staff for over twenty years. How many times did I use any of those three blocks on the streets?

The correct answer is none!

The training was out of the Home Office manual and never used by police officers. It was rubbish and not fit for purpose! For those who have ever been involved in a violent street fight (the type of fight a police officer is likely to face) you will know that it's often quick, energy sapping, sweaty, breathtaking, gritty, and often ends up in some sort of grapple on the floor. Not a place for choreographed playtime.

Fast forward to the issue of the modern-day, amazingly effective, metal, extendable, ASP-style baton. When we were issued with them it felt like 'day one' for a piece of kit which would be of real use to us. And it was. It even sounds like it means business as soon as you 'rack' it open and rest it on your shoulder ready for use. There's one command from the instructor for this piece of kit.

'If you have to use it, hit them as hard as you can.'

Simple. Effective. Just like the tips, tools, and techniques in this book.

Footnote: During training, officers are advised to avoid hitting 'red areas' – the head – because of the potential for serious injury or death and amber areas – joints – where a strike could result in life-changing injuries. Green areas are the 'preferred' target areas – the muscular parts of the arms and legs – being less likely to result in long-lasting or serious trauma.

The wooden staff was only good for breaking car windows to rescue babies accidentally locked in or overheated dogs in summer, or to smash a pain of glass to get into a house to save someone in trouble. Pretty much useless for what it was designed to do. Much like personal resilience training was back then, almost non-existent and, what was available, not fit for purpose.

Huge progress has been made in personal resilience and mental health support for police officers and society as a whole. The issue of the ASP was 'day one' in a new era of police self-defence capability. I hope you embrace the content of this book and make it your day one: a new chapter of wellbeing for you.

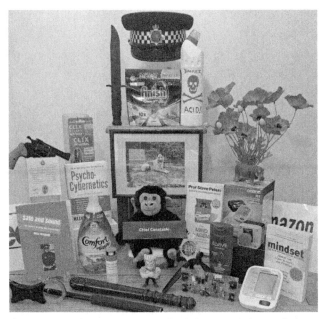

A selection of props, items and exhibits used during Safe and Sound training.

Mindset

Don't discount anything you read in here which you feel isn't for you. There is no 'one size fits all'. Some of the techniques won't be for you, and that's fine. All I ask is that you keep an open mind, try them out, see what works and, at the very least, keep them in your 'toolbox' ready to use in the future if you need to. You can store everything you read here, combine it with what you already know, add in your own story and experience, and hold the lot in your 'bank of brilliance' – your pot of good stuff ready to make a withdrawal whenever you need. Take the tips, tools, and techniques and use them to influence your character, mindset, and behaviour. Add them to things you already do, tweak them to make them fit your style. The stuff you read and already know will be a refresher. You will read things which are new to you and cause you suspicion! Remain open-minded in the knowledge that everything in this book is tried, tested, and proven to work by people operating in the toughest environments. Most of all, be proactive. Make working towards unshakeable personal resilience and strong mental health part of your life, turning what you learn into healthy habits woven into your life forever. Stay open-minded, open to opportunity, and open to learning.

The power of three

Nike will tell you to *Just do it*, Budweiser will remind you that theirs is the *King of Beers* and Sky TV encourages you to **Believe** *in Better*. The concept of using 'three' (in this case, three words) is used by the biggest companies in the world. Successful because it's simple and easy to remember, they stick in your mind and influence you to spend your hard-earned money on their products. This concept isn't new. Who can forget Mars Bars' promise to help you *Work, Rest and Play* since the 1950s and Rice Krispies have given you *Snap Crackle & Pop* in your breakfast cereal since 1928?

The power of three as a coaching and self-development tool works in a similar way. Successful because it's simple. Only three things to remember so it **feels** easy to do, meaning you're more likely to stick with it and gain maximum benefit. The power comes from combining three simple wellbeing tips, tools, or techniques **of your choice** (your own, from this book, or a combination) to deliver a big positive outcome of wellbeing support for you or the person you're helping. It is your choice. Easy to do, easy to remember, massive results. This simple approach is extremely effective and the best coaching tool I've ever used.

The Manchester Arena incident – a practical example

On 22 May 2017, the terrorist Salman Abedi walked into the foyer of the Manchester Arena and detonated a bomb he was carrying in his rucksack, killing 23 people and injuring hundreds more. The foyer had been packed with people leaving the arena having watched a concert by the pop star Ariana Grande. A catastrophic event which shook the communities of Manchester and beyond.

A massive police operation immediately sprang into action, and I'm proud to say my team was one of the first to respond.

For me as an operational police inspector, things changed literally overnight. Across the force everyone was put on twelve-hour shifts (as opposed to eight). All leave and rest days were cancelled and there was no opportunity to rest or decompress. By doing this, the force was able to maintain a 'normal' frontline police response (although it didn't feel anything like normal at the time) and release officers from frontline duties to start working on the huge and extremely complex investigation into the attack: gather evidence, search for suspects, support people affected, and bring offenders to justice.

My world became twelve-hour shifts performing a critical role as a police commander, with no days off. Additional responsibility as a wellbeing coach, supporting officers who were there on the night, supporting those who saved life and those who sadly couldn't, providing first point of contact for colleagues working on phone lines and in mortuaries. I sat with countless family liaison officers who, in turn, supported families who'd lost loved ones. I helped set up the Force Strategic Welfare Group and wrote the tactical plan to support the second largest police force in the country. I was busier than I'd ever been before, but who was looking after my welfare? Everything had become 'a priority' and there was no let-up in the pace of operations. My resilience was tested like never before, but I had to keep going. I believe, even to this day, that I got through those first six weeks by using the power of three. Three small changes to my routine, practised consistently every day changed my mindset and patterns of thinking in a positive way, boosted my energy, and provided an opportunity, albeit small, to reset every day and power me through. The three conscious choices I made were:

1. **Mindset** – I kept reminding myself that this was my time to really do some good and that although exhausting, the situation wouldn't last forever; I would get through and I would be OK. I repeated this numerous times throughout the day, sometimes in my head and sometimes out loud to myself. I never stopped believing this, and I always had hope that it would end. Some call these positive affirmations You'll will hear more about this in dog handler determination section later.

2. **Sleep** – I did a number of things to get the best quality sleep: regular early nights, no late-night telly, a bedtime routine to relax, and I cut out all alcohol for six weeks. Doing this gave me better quality sleep, more energy, and helped me feel fresher and better prepared to face the day. There's a whole section on sleep coming up!

3. **Reset** – I made sure I ran for at least twenty minutes on the treadmill at the police station every day. An opportunity to take a break and re energise. Oxygenate my body, shower, clean uniform on and back at it. Reset. Re-energised. Fresh and ready to go again. I'll show you various ways to 'reset' as we move forward through this book together.

Three simple things, practised consistently, helped get me through those tough times. A conscious decision and I knew it would work – of that, I had no doubt. I was going to get through and I was going to be OK, and I was! There is no reason why the power of three can't work exactly the same for you today!

The power of your personal story

You've heard a bit about my personal story earlier in the book, a snapshot in time and how this unique but painful experience was used to benefit others for many years during my service as a police officer. Your story is just as important. A unique mix of good, bad, and ugly. Even in our darkest days, there is light. Learning to be better next time. Recognition that we 'got through'; we are tougher, stronger, wiser than we were yesterday. Our life story is built on the stuff that happens to us day in and day out. [I wrote this during week five of the UK coronavirus lockdown. Everyone had their resilience tested during that period. Everyone was 'writing' their story. When you came out at the other end, how well did you reflect on your story?]   Did you choose to allow the change to daily life to grind you down? Did you reflect on the good stuff? How communities came together and supported each other? How you learned a new skill with what felt like 'extra' time on your hands? How you discovered ingenious new ways to connect with people? How you learned a new skill or took pleasure from seeing wildlife dominate our world. How will you use your story to lift you? How will you use your story to lift others? How will you capture the gold written into your own very personal and very unique story?

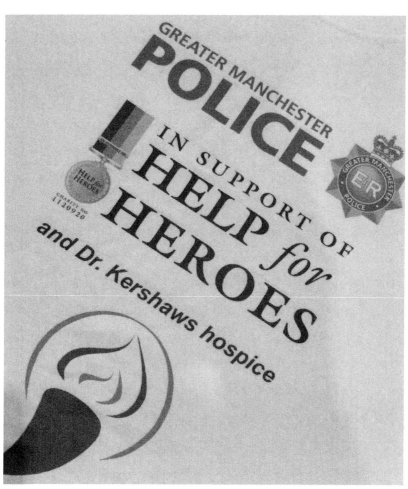

Giving back. One of the five ways to wellbeing and good for your soul.

Spokes – the more support you have, the stronger you will be

Spokes is a great analogy to demonstrate the benefits of having lots of different wellbeing tools in your toolbox. I demonstrate it on all my courses and have shared it hundreds of times with police officers and young people over the years. This is how it works.

Imagine yourself chatting with a friend or colleague and trying to make the case and at the same time drawing a circle on a piece of paper to represent a steel bicycle wheel. The wheel represents the other person. You draw just two spokes in the wheel. Each spoke representing one form of wellbeing. The fact that there are only two spokes used to signify minimal or limited wellbeing support to lean on. The analogy comes to life when you imagine the wheel with just a couple of spokes in it going over a little bump in the road (to signify the minor challenges we face every day). The wheel isn't very strong and the two spokes barely keeping it from wobbling. If the same wheel then goes over a big bump in the road (to signify a major life challenge such as a serious health diagnosis, death of a loved one, or other similar potentially catastrophic situation), we see the wheel buckle and crumble. If you then go on to draw loads more spokes in the wheel to strengthen it and equate those spokes to the tips, tools, and techniques in this book, for example, we see that the wheel – the person – becomes much stronger and better equipped not only to deal well with the small daily challenges we all face every day but also to be in a much stronger position to survive the big stuff when it hits.

A great analogy to aid learning and make the point. Used on my flipchart regularly and scribbled on countless bits of paper in police stations across Greater Manchester over the years!

The key message is to embrace as many tips, tools, and techniques as possible to increase the number of 'spokes' in your wheel, and using the tips, tools, and techniques in this book is a great way to stock up on your spokes!

Well, wobble and wipeout zones

These three words became common language in Greater Manchester Police and were used to 'check in' with people to get a sense of how they were. They fit with my concept of my power of three – three words, all beginning with W, which are easy to remember and add value to any wellbeing conversation or situation.

The following is my interpretation of the three zones.

The well zone – Life is going well. I'm engaged in meaningful work, I have purpose in my life, and I'm generally happy with my lot.

The wobble zone – I'm not as happy as I used to be. There are a few changes in my life which are unsettling me, things don't feel right, and aren't likely to get better anytime soon.

The wipeout zone – I've had enough. I feel burnt out and unhappy all the time. This situation isn't getting better, and I feel like I can't carry on.

On my course, I stress the importance of self-awareness and recognising when you start to dip out of the well zone and into the wobble zone. We all have 'off' days and it's absolutely OK to be not OK, but if that starts to happen more and more, and you start to dip down more often, you MUST do something about it. Speak to someone, lean on the stuff in this book, seek some support from your network, get out into nature and breathe, immerse yourself in stuff that makes you feel good, whatever works for you, but you MUST take action to restore the balance and get yourself moving back towards the well zone. Doing nothing is NOT an option!

The concept of well, wobble and wipeout is primarily used as a tool for individuals but can also be used to sense check an organisation and is useful when going through change processes to assess staff wellbeing during the journey. For the purposes of this book, however, we will stick with individual use, your own, where you ask the question of yourself, or where you ask the person sitting opposite when trying to get a handle on how they are. There are two main options for use:

You ask the question: 'Whereabouts do you think you are you on this line?' and draw a line on a sheet of paper with the three words spaced out, marking the line with an X to signify their own self-assessment. This will give you a starting point and something to work with and can be followed up with questions like:

- What can I do to support you and help you move up the scale? (It might be that **at this time,** just to listen with intent to understand is all that's needed with no need to try to find solutions.)

- What could you do to help move yourself up the scale one notch? (Quite often, you or the person you're supporting knows what needs to happen next and this question is particularly powerful because it empowers the other person.)

The key message here is about emotional intelligence and self-awareness, in yourself and others. It's about recognising what's 'normal' and noticing the point when you move from the well zone into the wobble zone and doing something about it before things get out of hand.

Marks out of ten

This is a simple technique which is gaining traction in the world of mental health support and fits brilliantly into any wellbeing plan as a self-assessment tool. It's grounded in emotional intelligence, specifically self-awareness, knowing what's right for you, what's normal, and what's not, and it's a slightly different technique to the one above.

You take all the factors in your life during a normal time (if there is such a thing!) and add them together. How you feel normally, your happiness, sense of purpose, job satisfaction, health, finances, social networks, relationships, work/home life balance, basically everything about your life added together during a normal time and give yourself a mark out of ten. For me, that would be around a seven or an eight. I go up to nine or ten when I'm delivering my Safe and Sound courses because that's something I'm passionate about and I love it, but I'm not on cloud nine every day and normally sit at eight because I'm fairly happy with my lot.

The gold from this technique is recognising when I dip down more than three points. Maybe a blip in a relationship, a financial worry or health concern, it can be anything. I'm going to be OK with dipping down for a day or two, again, OK to be not OK, but I'm very aware if I dip down for a longer period, and I will take action to bring myself up. I will lean on my spokes, I will speak to a trusted friend, I will flood my life with things which make me happy, and I will pay more attention to my own self-care to bring me back up the scale. Super simple to do, the key message is, again, about self-awareness and noticing and, just as importantly, taking action and doing something about it. I lean on my support network when I need to, but I never forget that my first responsibility is for me to take action and do something myself!

This is another technique I found very useful to support police officers, and I highly recommend it to readers who manage people as a way to open up conversations about wellbeing.

Give it a try and let me know how you get on.

Triggers

Trigger is the word I use to describe those things which make you 'go off'. Like a trigger being pulled on a gun. The things that wind you up, make you grit your teeth and clench your fists. The things that bug you, annoy you, irritate you, and make you do and say things you might not normally do or say.

Brought to life during my workshops where delegates are invited to hold, examine and 'play' with a real firearm, something most people never get the opportunity to do. This exercise always generates healthy discussion about all sorts of things and highlights the point. Triggers. Do you know what yours are? Are you aware how much your words and behaviour change when your trigger is pulled? Are the changes good or bad? Do you notice a change in your behaviour before it's pulled? What do you do? Are you able to control your thoughts and feelings or do you allow them to control you? The exercise generates a whole load of questions all connected to emotional awareness and intelligent thinking and, as you read, I encourage you to reflect on this.

A wide range of examples are shared. Poor driving is always in there. Road rage is a likely topic for discussion. It's a good one too, many crashes, assaults, and even murder have resulted from a seemingly minor driving indiscretion. Someone's not said thank you after being 'let out' of a junction, resulting in aggressive hand signals, swearing, loss of control, and violence in the middle of the road, leading to a ruined day!

Bad manners always irritate people:

> There's no excuse for bad manners, people not saying please and thank you.

As the facilitator standing at the front, I observe the contributors' body language and reflect it back to them to see whether they're aware of their change in behaviour as they recount an experience of someone's bad manners.

Think tone of voice, hardened jawline, crossed arms, or clenched fists. Often, they're not aware and feel embarrassed at having this, gently and kindly, pointed out to them. It's not about embarrassment; it is about self-awareness and learning.

Triggers can come from anywhere. We are all different and what bugs one person won't bug another. Similarly, triggers change with age, life experience, demographics and where we are in life. The learning point here is remembering that AND noticing the changes in us as a result.

In every session I do there are some, let's say, 'a little out of the ordinary' triggers shared by people.

'I can't stand the way my dad eats – he even eats salad noisily.'

'He can't load the dishwasher properly. I've told him a thousand times and still he gets it wrong.'

'The way my other half wees loudly when he's in the toilet winds me right up.'

I've just noticed all of these examples involve men. Does this wind you up?

For me, it's bad manners. Specifically, people who cough and sneeze in the air. I hate it with a passion. Its rude, disgusting, unhygienic, and shows a complete disregard for people in the area. Can you tell it's one of my triggers by the words I write? (And this was before the pandemic hit!)

Get to know your triggers, what winds you up, makes you grit your teeth and clench your fists. Self-awareness, emotional intelligence, knowing yourself. Notice when these things happen and feelings begin to rise in a bad way and do something about it to help you respond well rather than react badly to whatever's going on.

The sneezing superintendent

I worked at Greater Manchester Police Headquarters for four years and was privileged to support some new and exciting training and development projects for front line officers.

It was an office type role. White shirt and tie, smartly pressed dress uniform trousers and shoes with 'bulled' (highly polished) toe caps. Very smart attire, unlike the all-black military style uniform and boots worn by 'operational' cops which is often described as 'military looking' but much more practical for working on the front line.

The role attracted nicknames from the real grafters outside on the front line: 'shiny arse' (because you sat at a computer all day wearing out the seat of your trousers and making them shine) or 'plastics' (a term used to signify you weren't a real police officer because you worked inside all the time). Nevertheless, it was a very enjoyable time for me, a nice break from front-line work, and as I was working directly with the Force Command team, it gave me the opportunity to see how the force operated from a higher level, which is always interesting.

Headquarters has lots of senior officers, or bosses as they're known affectionately, working there, making the big decisions which come running the second largest police force in the UK. Many vying for importance, milling around in a haze of ego-induced self-importance as they bustled around from meeting to meeting. The building itself was new and very smart. Open plan areas with breakout rooms on every one of its six floors to hold private meetings, canteens on every floor, a restaurant and lifts that worked! It was a lovely place to work.

I was sitting at my open plan desk, on the fourth floor, surrounded by other open plan desks occupied by people working in an open-planned way (get the picture?). Mr Henshaw, a superintendent and three ranks above me, worked near us. He was a man full of his own self-importance, one of the more senior ranks on the floor and not averse to a spot of bullying in his spare time. He had also developed an irritating cough.

On the day in question, he walked past my open plan working space and, without covering his mouth, let out a rattly, throaty cough as he walked past me. I had a horrible image of spit and green phlegm flying into the air and felt my hackles stand up. Ten minutes later, having exited his tremendously important meeting, he headed back past me again and let rip another cough, right next to me, no attempt to cover it up, straight up into the air. My blood pressure was rising but I was still not quite brave enough to stand up and say anything. I looked around at my team. I knew they were thinking the same. The look on my face must have told them exactly what I was thinking, and they weren't pleasant thoughts!

Well, it doesn't take a genius to guess what happened next. Half an hour later, he walks past my desk again, cough, splutter and full-on sneezes into the air!

Now, I don't know whether this has happened to you. Your body starts moving and doing things and your mouth starts to chuck words out that everybody can hear at exactly the same time as your sensible brain is saying to sit down and shut up. Too late: my 'trigger' has been well and truly pulled!

'I'm not being funny sir!' I say in an angry, sarcastic tone, 'I don't want to catch your cold, and I'm fairly sure my team don't want it either.' What a hero!

Don't be fooled into thinking this is 'something and nothing'. It might be 'outside' the police service where rank and egos might not matter as much, but this was different. This was the 'legend' (in his own mind) the great Superintendent Henshaw who'd been humiliated and given some home truths in front of 40 or 50 colleagues, all of whom (on a rank scale) were subordinate to him.

My tone of voice whilst espousing my wisdom was gruff. Not normally how a sergeant would address a superintendent.

He stopped, I slunk back into my chair, heart pounding (yes, really) a glare lasting a few seconds and then off he went without a murmur. Did he say anything? No, he didn't. Did he hold it against me? Who knows, suffice to say I was promoted shortly after and returned to the front line and our paths never crossed again. Do I regret it? Not one bit, but a good example of my 'trigger' being pulled and the reaction that followed.

I could have dealt with it differently, and hindsight is a great teacher. I should have recognised a finger was on the trigger because I hate people coughing into the air. He'd done it twice already and my hackles were raised. I should have acted then, moved away, gone for a walk, or asked him to come into a side room so I could have a 'chat' with him. It would have been the more professional thing to do. My trigger, in that moment, decided otherwise.

The stress bucket

What if you have several triggers and they all get pulled one after the other? How do we cope with that?

A good way to picture this and describe it if you're supporting someone else is the analogy of the stress bucket.

Imagine a see-through plastic bucket. The bucket represents you. Imagine it being filled with water. The water represents stress pouring into you from different directions. As each trigger is pulled and more stress is added to your life, a bit more water goes into the bucket until the point where it reaches the top. This is the critical point: you can't take any more and it overflows. It's the 'straw that broke the camel's back', the end of the road, you've had enough, you've entered the wipe-out zone.

An analogy I've used hundreds of times to support police officers who are sitting in front of me and stressed. I draw the bucket on a piece of paper, explain the concept of it filling up and draw this. Doing so helps to move their attention from an emotional state and help them engage the computer brain, the part of the brain that deals with logic. It's simple, it makes sense, it calms people down and helps them understand what's going on. From there we move to 'What are we going to do to fix this?'

In our day-to-day lives, the bucket fills and empties all the time. The trick is to keep it draining, draining the stress out of your life. Engaging tips, tools, techniques, and strategies which keep the tap open to let the water constantly drain out to help you decompress. The tips tools and techniques in this book will all help keep that tap open.

I'm late

You've got an important meeting at work this morning, but you've not been sleeping too well recently. You don't hear the alarm and oversleep. The first cupful cascades into the bucket and you're already starting the day on the back foot. You're running late. You rush to get up and your mind is already beginning to race. You will be moving into heavier traffic because you got up late and this means you are 'on the last minutes' for work. Your bucket is beginning to fill.

You race out of the house into the car and put your foot down; a near miss with another car because your mind is racing and you're not concentrating fully plunges a cupful in. Did that speed camera flash? Doesn't matter whether it did or didn't, the fact you're thinking about it has added another cup to the bucket. You scream up to the security barrier at work but there's a queue at the gate to get past security. If only you'd been ten minutes earlier, you'd have missed the queue and be in drinking coffee. Water trickles in as you queue. You check your messages and see your daughter asking where her trainers are for her sports lesson. Add one large cupful. You're fuming because you told her to get her stuff ready last night and she chose to ignore your instruction. One large cup – in it goes, from height! (In any case, what does she expect me to do about it right now?)

Into the office and grab a coffee.

With seconds to spare, you dash through the door to find the meeting in full flow. You're late. 'I emailed everybody this morning – did you not see it?' asks the boss.

It's not yet hit ten o'clock in the morning and your bucket is already close to overflowing.

Let's replay this with some bucket emptying tips, tools, and techniques added in **bold**.

You start the day on the back foot. You're already running late. You rush to get up and your mind is already beginning to race, you will be moving into heavier traffic because you got up late and this is likely to make you 'on the last minutes' for work.

Slow your breathing down. This will still allow you to move quickly but also help keep you in control of your thinking, so you think and behave rationally. The bucket is beginning to empty.

You race out of the house into the car and put your foot down, a near miss with another car due to not concentrating fully. **Mindful driving. Concentrate on the moment, not what's just happened; that moment's gone.** The bucket is emptying because you changed your thinking.

Did that speed camera flash? **It's been and gone; it's outside your control at that moment. Forget it (for now). The fact that** you've dealt well with the issue means no more water has been added to your bucket.

You manage to get to work on time but there's a queue at the gate to get past security. **Recognising that this is out of your control will prevent water going in. Slowing your breathing and practising mindfulness will drain it.**

You check your messages and see you daughter asking where her trainers are for sports lesson **Out of your control, let it go, a valuable life lesson for your daughter and this will not be important in six months' time. Let it go.**

Into the office, grab a coffee. At last, ready to go with seconds to spare. **You walk towards the meeting room, slowing your breathing; slowing your physiology will keep you calm and composed, ready to respond well to anything thrown at you. Your bucket has been emptying. You've got space in there and you're in a strong position. Celebrate your wins from the last hour.**

You dash through the door to find the meeting in full flow. You're late. **This is not a problem for you. You have space in your bucket and have arrived in complete control. You apologise for being late, calmly take your seat and focus in the moment on what needs to be done.**

There are sections in this book dedicated to each of the tips, tools, and techniques highlighted.

This is just one hypothetical but realistic example to demonstrate how to use the techniques in this book to turn on the tap and drain the stress from your bucket. It also highlights the need to practise what you learn here. This is critical so that they 'kick in' when you need them most. The more you know, the more you practise, the better these tips, tools, and techniques will serve you.

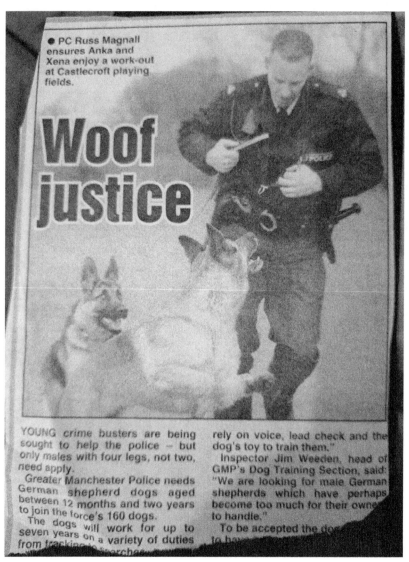

● PC Russ Magnall ensures Anka and Xena enjoy a work-out at Castlecroft playing fields.

Woof justice

YOUNG crime busters are being sought to help the police – but only males with four legs, not two, need apply.

Greater Manchester Police needs German shepherd dogs aged between 12 months and two years to join the force's 160 dogs.

The dogs will work for up to seven years on a variety of duties from tracking to searches.

rely on voice, lead check and the dog's toy to train them."

Inspector Jim Weeden, head of GMP's Dog Training Section, said: "We are looking for male German shepherds which have perhaps become too much for their owners to handle."

To be accepted the dog

Time to play! Even police dogs need timeout to decompress.

Practice

One of the things I enjoy most from providing personal resilience support is that I learn something new from every workshop I do. I go to great lengths to try to explain that although I'm standing at the front of the room delivering the session, I'm not an expert, and it isn't about dictating or telling you how you should build personal resilience, far from it. I try to make the case for you to treat your own personal resilience like a dental or doctors' practice. A specialism which grows and gets better all the time. When you adopt this approach, you see that you don't just read a book or go on a course and suddenly you are super resilient! It's a slow burn. A combination of tips, tools, techniques, and knowledge all wrapped up in your story.

My job is to share what I've learned with you. If you see, read, or experience something you think will serve you well, have it, if not, that's fine. It's possible that you'll read stuff in here which completely switches you off, and that's fine too. You do what works for you. All I ask is that you consider what you read here and reflect on how it might support you, either as it's delivered by me or by you adapting, tweaking, and moulding to fit your character, style, and need.

I urge you to commit to your own personal resilience practice which grows stronger every day. For my own practice, I read, reflect, watch TEDX clips on YouTube and observe people around me. I try new things to see what works and what doesn't, can I adapt it or try a different approach, in other words, what can I learn? I have a growth mindset and above all else – I PRACTISE.

CHAPTER 2

Networks

During the coronavirus lockdown of 2020, people were asked to stay at home, protect the NHS, and save lives. (Power of three on a grand scale right there!) Overnight, people's support networks were dramatically reduced, and we had to find ingenious ways to connect with each other. Social media sprang into life with communities connecting by messaging and video calling. I did too. Since retiring from the police, although I've not stopping working, I had been connecting with (well, going to the pub with!) ex-police dog handlers who I'd worked with over the years, who, like me, were finding their way through new chapters in their lives outside policing. We meet once a month in a country pub, check in with each other, swap war stories, have a few drinks and a lot of laughs, and I look forward to it a lot.

This is the stuff that keeps your spirits up, no surprise in any of that. When, suddenly, thanks to this pesky virus, it was taken away, I missed the human connection, like we all did. I missed seeing them. A stark reminder that anything can be taken away in an instant and it pays to be grateful for what we have, but more about gratitude later. Thanks to social media, specifically WhatsApp, we formed an online group and began chatting, sharing jokes, letting each other know what we were up to, having banter and generally keeping each other's spirits up. Exactly what we did as serving police officers for 30 years.

The virus created an opportunity to place a lens fairly and squarely onto this group to see why it worked so well and why it was so effective in helping us all remain resilient. Well, one thing it's not is a bunch of individuals who are very alike (except for our love of dogs and support for law and order!). No, we are a bunch of misfits really. Dog handlers are often described as an odd bunch when they're 'in the job'. They're often dirty, covered in mud, don't do paperwork very well and struggle with interviews. They are, however, particularly good at what they do. They give good advice and have outstanding ability to make good decisions. They don't seem odd to me at all! We are a group of mixed ages. Some are properly retired, some are still working, we've got ex-Royal Navy, ex-shopkeepers, ex-engineers, some are loaded, and some are skint! Yes, an odd bunch with mixed interests and very differing ideas about just about any topic you choose! So, what draws us together? Why does it work so well? How does this network support resilience, and what can we learn from it?

Well, for starters, we have a shared history: we've 'been there and done it.' Every one of us understands the fear of being in the middle of a field in the middle of the night with only your police dog for support, facing some of Manchester's most violent individuals. Each of us, because of our shared history, has credibility.

Choose people for your network who are credible and honest. As a bunch, we all have something to offer and have an opinion about everything, but it's more than that: these dog handlers are straight talking. If something's not right, they will tell you, and everyone should have those honest, straight talkers in their tribe!

Choose people for your network who are reliable. When the s**t hits the fan, I know that I can rely on any one of them to come to my aid and help me out. Period.

Choose people for your network who will lift you up and not drag you down. Building networks includes workplaces, families (although it's hard to choose your family, you're stuck with what you're given there!) and personal relationships. Think about your 'go-to people'. Are they loyal, trustworthy, dependable? Do they provide good advice even if it's not advice you want to hear? Do they lift you, encourage you, push you forward, and give you hope? These are the people you want around you.

Recognise that this is a proactive thing, you build your network and constantly review who's wrapped around you supporting you. It's important to remember that your network will change throughout your life. Some people will stay forever, and some won't. Don't waste your time or energy on anyone who's toxic or drags you down – they have to go! My support network who helped me pass police promotion assessments are not the same as those who support me now as a resilience coach. It's worth giving it some thought and reflecting whether your network could do with an overhaul. If it could, act!

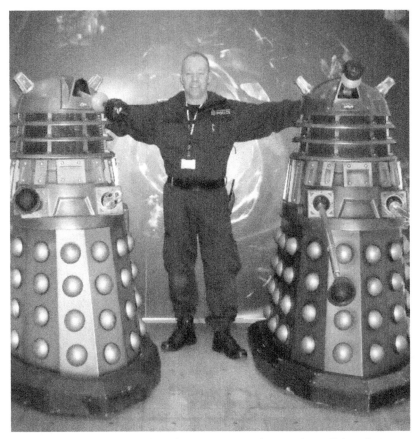

Never underestimate the value of a strong network around you. Taken during an overnight counter terrorist search at Media City Salford.

Blood pressure

I mentioned from the outset that this book is more concerned with the mind and the way we think about things than with physical exercise in terms of supporting resilience, and that remains the case. You already know that physical exercise, even twenty minutes a day, is good for you in terms of building resilience, reducing stress, and improving your overall wellbeing. There is one element of physical health I want to share with you, though, and that's the dangers of salt in your diet. Specifically, how excess salt raises blood pressure and can lead to heart attacks, strokes, and early death. It is described as a hidden killer and because of this it features in my workshops, and here's why.

Monday afternoons at one o'clock were an event for all inspectors. This was the weekly performance meeting at the divisional HQ. An opportunity to come together with senior leaders to check how everyone was doing to protect our communities and keep people safe. Police, council, pubs and clubs, and various children's services were all represented, and as long as crime wasn't out of control on your patch and you had effective plans in place, the meetings weren't difficult. These meetings provided an opportunity to chat informally with all the other inspectors on the division before the main meeting got underway. Generally a light-hearted affair and a chance to catch up and engage in some cheerful banter.

At midday I walked into the police station in good time for the meeting and plenty of opportunity to chat beforehand. As a creature of habit, I walked to the inspector's desk. A plain desk in the corner of the open plan ground floor, located right next to the sergeants' desks with a commanding view of the whole floor to keep an eye on things.

As I approached, I saw the morning inspector sitting behind the desk. A ruddy faced Irishman, competent, witty, with a fierce temper when roused. He greeted me with a bemused expression on his face as he saw me staring down at a portable blood pressure testing machine perched on the table next to his computer with the expandable cuff fixed firmly around the bicep of his left arm.

'What's that for?' I asked curiously. 'I've got high blood pressure,' he replied. 'The doctor's told me to take five readings a day, at intervals, and make a note of the results so he can keep an eye on how I'm doing.'

To hear him say he had high blood pressure didn't surprise me. He was quite visibly overweight. By his own admission, he didn't do as much exercise as he should and drank too much whiskey. He was a single man who liked his single malt. By this time, the other inspectors had arrived and were all milling around the desk, watching this spectacle unfold and flitting between asking serious questions and making fun of him. It got the better of me. 'Can I have a go?' Typical cop. Typical lad. He's got a 'toy' and I want a go!

Now this request was fuelled by a large slice of arrogance. I'm thinking to myself that my blood pressure would be good. I keep fit, stopped smoking over 20 years ago, have a fairly good diet and my stress levels are low (I am the resilience coach after all!). I'm bound to be OK and can show all my peers how healthy I am. I was extremely confident all would be well as I fixed the cuff onto my left bicep and pressed 'start'. A slow hum from the machine, the cuff expanded and gripped my bicep before slowly deflating and delivering the numerical results on the monitor. I remember smiling in anticipation…

Not only were the numbers high, but the orange warning lamp also lit up on the dashboard indicating hypertension, in other words – high blood pressure! 'Can't be right,' I exclaimed. 'This machine must be faulty.' (The arrogance continues.) I decided to change arms and try again, much to the amusement of my peers. Of course, the machine wasn't faulty, and my ego was brought down to earth with a bump. I walked up the stairs and into the meeting although my mind wasn't concentrating on anything other than what had just happened and that orange light.

It frightened me.

Later that week I booked in to see the nurse at my doctors' surgery where it was confirmed that, although I was generally healthy, I did have high blood pressure. After answering loads of health-related questions, the nurse gave me my results.

'You eat too much salt. It's killing you slowly, may lead to heart disease or a stroke and will almost certainly contribute to you getting diabetes.'

'But salt? How come?' I thought.

I had salt on everything. I loved salt, every meal almost. I'd come out of the gym and eat chicken and pasta with salt on. My snack of choice was salted peanuts, and I had to eat the whole pack. Chippy tea Fridays were a meal to look forward to: 'Salt and vinegar, love?' 'Yes please.' Then I'd take it all home for my family and put more salt on mine because there wasn't enough on for me. You get the picture.

I will never forget the nurse's final comment as my consultation concluded and I was putting my coat on.

'Too much salt can kill you. It's a silent killer and not enough people know how bad it can be for them.' Those words still haunt me today.

I share the story with you. The story features in all my workshops. Will you help me spread the message? After all, what use is resilience if you drop dead because you weren't aware? Sobering thought, isn't it?

Soak time

It was February 2005. I'd been working on the Oldham division of Greater Manchester Police for three years and had found my feet at the rank of sergeant having been promoted three years earlier. I needed something new to challenge me. One of the benefits of being a police officer is the diversity of roles you can specialise in, and I was looking for that challenge at the same time the divisional bulletin came out in February that year.

WANTED!

OFFICERS REQUIRED FOR EXCITING NEW OPPORTUNITY TO JOIN

SPECIALIST SEARCH TEAM.

PLEASE APPLY WITH A SHORT REPORT DETAILING WHY YOU SHOULD BE CONSIDERED FOR THIS ROLE.

That was more than enough for me. Exciting. New opportunity. Search. Sold as seen! I applied, passed the interview and, together with six constables also specially selected, attended at the force training academy, Sedgley Park, Prestwich in Manchester. Now this was no ordinary course. Generally, in the police you are supported, encouraged, coached, and mentored to pass practically any course you do. This was quite different. It was being run by the army, and not just any branch of the army: this was bomb disposal, or Explosive Ordnance Disposal to give it its proper name. The course was pass or fail, and it was made crystal clear that if we didn't excel, we would be off the course and returned to division. There was no place for second best. Only the highest standards would be accepted. I loved it.

As promised, the course was tough, and we were put through our paces. We were given the latest intelligence updates to help us understand the national and international threat level. We were given demonstrations of the power of different explosive devices and the carnage they can cause. We handled and got to know inside out numerous bombs (improvised explosive devices) and their component parts. We were taught to search in a methodical, logical manner to ensure nothing, and I mean nothing, was missed during the many practical searches we did where training items were hidden for us to find, all under the watchful eye of our instructors, ammunition technical officers or ATOs as they are known. These are men and women who know their stuff having honed their skills in Bosnia, Iraq, Afghanistan, and Northern Ireland. They expected us to get it right and gave us short shrift if we got anything wrong. I was in awe of these soldiers – I'm not afraid to say that out loud. Brave professional people who have done it at the sharp end. I wanted my team and I to get things right, to honour them, their commitment, and what they stood for.

I will never forget our instructor, a sergeant nearing the end of his military career, talking about his experiences in Northern Ireland. About donning the 'big suit', the huge protective blast suit designed to protect the soldier if a bomb goes off near them. I will never forget the silence in my team as he talked about doing the 'long walk' towards a car packed with explosives. An empty street. Just him and the car. He did this many times and thankfully survived to tell us the story. Many of his friends and colleagues did not.

Normally, and prior to donning the suit and doing the long walk, ATOs will use a piece of kit called a wheelbarrow: a robot, white in colour nowadays with wheels, but green and with tracks, like a tank, in days gone by. These are an incredible piece of kit. Remote controlled and bristling with equipment. Their job is to take the place of the soldier, approach the IED or suspect vehicle, briefcase, container, or package, and shoot it, touch it, move it, blast water at high pressure at it, basically perform one or more tasks so the soldiers don't have to. The wheelbarrows during the Northern Ireland conflict were often seen firing at the door locks of vehicles to a) get in the vehicle or b) disrupt the vehicle in some way to damage the explosive device or its component parts enough so that it didn't explode. The wheelbarrows saved countless lives. Better that a replaceable piece of machinery takes the force of any explosion than a human.

The ATOs call the time immediately after the disruption 'soak time' time to see what, if anything, happens and whether the IED will blow up. It also gives them time to think about their strategy and what they will do next.

Soak time has a direct link to resilience and can be an incredible personal resilience tool.

Think about it like this. How many times have you seen someone react badly, immediately after something is said or they see something? Think road rage whilst driving. Think the one punch in a pub which kills someone. Think a caustic nasty comment to your partner because you're tired and irritable. Almost all these behaviours are driven by emotions. We're back to emotional intelligence and the fact that our emotions, if we don't control them, have the potential to control us and wreck our lives in an instant. If the ATO allows soak time for things to settle before deciding what to do next, why can't we? A skill which will help you respond well rather than react badly to whatever situation or challenge you face, and it's not hard to do if you practise. Practise, and embed it into your flinch response, so ingrained in your character that you do it automatically when you need it.

The first element to nailing this one is emotional awareness. When is stuff like this likely to happen to you? What winds you up, pulls your trigger, stresses you out, and makes you lose your cool? (Incidentally, this technique works just as well when you are blindsided by something completely unexpectedly and out of the blue.) You have to practise to **recognise** what's going on, that's the emotional intelligence/awareness bit. Notice how your behaviour may change as a result. You must practise this technique to make it second nature. I repeat this bit because it's so important! The second element is soak time. Create some space, stop talking or ask questions, listen more, take a break, allow silence, walk away, practise the breathing tips I share with you, reset. Do **something** to create soak time. Space. To help you respond well, rather than react badly.

Paula and Rick

I was sharing this technique with a group of female ex-prisoners, all of whom had attended the 'school of hard knocks'. They taught me loads about resilience. That's the beauty of this work: every course I run, I learn something new. Anyway, I'd just reached the end when one of the ladies, 'Paula', put her hand up. She went on to tell a tale about something which had happened to her two months ago and she wished now that she'd known about soak time.

Paula had received a text message from her friend 'Karen' saying that Paula's boyfriend, 'Rick', was sitting with another women having coffee in in the town centre. As far as Paula knew, Rick was supposed to be at work. There were gasps from the others in the room. I think we all started to make immediate assumptions. Paula and Rick had been going through a rocky patch, he was drinking too much, money was tight, and they'd been arguing a lot. On top of this, Rick had a nasty temper and would fly off the handle at the slightest thing. The pressure on their relationship was mounting.

Rick walked through the front door that night to a punch in the face from Paula. In Paula's words, 'All hell broke loose.' They fought, screamed, the kids were crying, the police arrived. Rick was arrested for assault. As is often the case when emotions settle, the truth and detail come out and things are not always as they first seem. People can behave rationally, always the best option. Rick, throughout, maintained that he loved her; he hadn't been seeing 'another woman' in that sense but had been seeing a counsellor and that's who he was meeting on the day in question in the town centre. He knew his ability to control his anger was causing huge issues in their relationship and was affecting everything else, his drinking, finances, and work.

The counsellor had been supporting him, free of charge, having been provided by the charity Victim Support to help him control his anger. He did not want his anger issues to end their relationship. He did want to control it and surprise Paula by turning his life round, curbing his drinking, and, ultimately, asking Paula to marry him. The story had been checked and verified by the police. Rick was telling the truth.

Soak time. Find a way to let emotions settle so that you're able to respond well, rather than react badly. If only Paula had allowed soak time. If only Paula had asked questions. If only Paula hadn't made assumptions. If only Paula had stuck to the facts. If only Paula had taken rescue breaths as Rick walked through the door. If only Paula had created soak time. If only. We can all be guilty of that.

Overthinking

If you were to ask me what has the biggest negative impact on my own wellbeing, it would be this: I'm a natural worrier. I remember being a newly promoted sergeant, and one Friday night, my new boss, the inspector, popped her head round the door to my office and wished me a good weekend before walking off saying that she needed to speak to me about something on Monday morning. Most people wouldn't have given that a second thought, but not me. I worried about it all weekend. Have I done something wrong? Is it a complaint? Should I be worried? Do I need to prepare? What is it? My mind played loads of different scenarios over and over on a loop. It even affected the quality of my sleep. Of course, Monday morning came and the issue she wanted to talk about was nowhere near as bad as I'd imagined. All that worry, overthinking, and wasted time and emotional energy. Not good for anyone. Overthinking can hit us at any time. An unclear text message with loads of gaps which our brain, logically, tries to fill with guesses and assumptions. An overheard conversation where you only get a bit of the tale and start second-guessing the rest. A health diagnosis which immediately spins you out of control and straight into worst-case scenarios and that's before we start on families and relationships! Overthinking, like worrying about things outside your control, will steal your time and sap your emotional energy. My tips to make sure this doesn't happen to you are really simple and I do this every day.

- Become more self-aware and pay more attention to when this starts to creep in. Notice the situations when it's likely to happen so you catch it and stop it snowballing out of control. Even if something happens out of the blue, this technique will still work.
- Follow the learning from interview training for detectives and **stick to the facts**. No guessing, no assumptions, no filling in the spaces with what might have happened: **stick to the facts.**
- Train yourself to think like this so when you notice yourself starting to overthink you immediately and consciously bring your thoughts back to the mantra **stick to the facts; what's the reality here?**

You then go on to adopt the power of three, add in some soak time and breath work, and you're on to a winner. Calming your mind, calming your emotions, and creating space to come back to logical thought to respond well, rather than react badly. If only Paula had known this. How differently things might have turned out for her and Rick.

A personal example where this worked for me was when I noticed a mole on my torso had changed colour, size, and texture. Changes which healthcare professionals tell us need to be checked out to rule out cancer.

Me now (sticking to the facts)

- I've got a mole.
- It's changed.
- It's vital I get it checked out.

That's it.

Me the overthinker

- I've got a mole.
- It's changed.
- I must have cancer, have I got cancer? I must have, I'm going online to read, I'm in the right age bracket to get cancer so it must be, should I get it checked out? Do I want to know? Early diagnosis and all that, I might just leave it, it'll go away, no it won't, what if it doesn't? But I don't want to know, I'm scared, am I going to die? it will be, it must be...

I got it checked out. It was a normal sign of ageing and nothing else.

Got it?

Dog handler determination

We can all be guilty of 'selling ourselves short' when it comes to what the experts call 'inner dialogue'. Put simply, the stuff we tell ourselves. Maybe this has happened to you. Maybe you've seen someone lose out because they told themselves that they weren't 'good enough' or they'll 'never be able to do it' or didn't go for that job or promotion because 'someone else is bound to be better qualified'. A negative influence on us often stemming from childhood experience.

Negative self-talk can be a self-fulfilling prophecy; you tell yourself you can't and as a result you don't. It all links together. I was privileged to have the role of police dog handler for nine years. Probably the best nine years of my service and a dream job for me since being a young lad. The bond you develop with your dog is so strong and the feelings you get when you catch criminals is off the scale. Working with my dog developed what I call 'dog handler determination' and it links very well to the topic were talking about here. This is how it works.

If my police colleagues call for us as a dog team to go through the door and deal with a high level of threat – someone holding a hostage at knifepoint, a maniac armed with a firearm, or a crazy brandishing a baseball bat – they are relying on us. They need us to show up for them, protect them, and do a good job. Often, we are their last line of defence. I feel this, and that weight of responsibility weighs heavily on my mind, but in a good way: I use it to spur me on.

The public expect me to be there for them. They pay me well, rely on me, and trust me to do a good job for them. That responsibility weighs heavily on my mind, but in a good way, and I use it to fuel me and push me on. I choose to think like that, and I'm determined to do a good job. I will not let them down. I can still feel the determination as I type…

I know police dog training in Greater Manchester Police is the best in the world. My canine companion and I have been through sixteen weeks of initial training. We learned together and are a perfect fit. I love my dog more than I love some members of my own family, and she loves me. She would die for me, and rightly or wrongly, I would do the same for her. We are inseparable professionals. That bond is like superglue. Add all this together and I have a pretty potent combination of thoughts, beliefs, experience, power, grit, and determination driving me forward. She won't let me down and I will never let her down.

I approach the door, dog snarling, heart pounding, and adrenaline rushing through my veins. My mindset at this point is set, galvanised by all my beliefs and thoughts as the final piece of the jigsaw slots into place as we go through the door...

There is only going to be one winner here … and it is going to be us!.

This is dog handler determination.

This approach served me well for nine years as a dog handler and continues to serve me well today, even though my challenges are different now. We never failed. Sure, we got some bumps, bruises, cuts, and scrapes over the years (just like we all do in life) but the unwavering belief in what we had to do served us well.

You have your own dog handler determination; we all do. It's just a matter of looking inside you to see what matters to you. What do you stand for? Who do you love? Who are you fighting for? What makes your heart sing? What are your passions in life, your successes, the challenges you've overcome? What about your beliefs? Get a notepad, start writing, start tapping into all your good memories and use them to feed your chatter. Imagine a flame deep inside your belly: what is it that's going to turn it up? What are the things in your life that inspire, motivate, and fire you up? Think about the tough times and how you got through. It might not have been pretty and might have been painful, but you did it, you're on it, you're winning. Use your experience to stoke your flame. Develop your own mantra, your own pattern of thinking, your own words of wisdom you can tap into anytime to spur you on. It doesn't matter who you are, what stage in life you're at, we can all do this. It is a learnable, coachable, trainable thing and it will serve you well, every day of your life. A steely determination to never give up needs to be part of your practice.

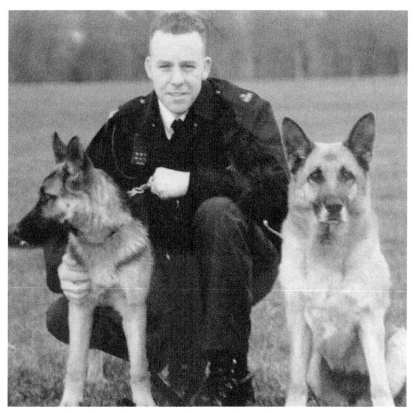

My Police dogs: Anka (looking at the camera) and Xena, the inspiration for 'dog handler determination'

See it

Visualisation is the ability to see a successful ending to a task or challenge in your mind's eye. It's a mental picture of you crashing through the tape in first place and holding the trophy aloft in front of cheering crowds, picking up your certificates and seeing the pride in the faces of your family. It's opening the letter and seeing the words 'Congratulations, we'd be delighted to offer you the position' or taking a bow at the end of a fantastic presentation with huge sense of satisfaction washing over you. You see it, feel it, taste it. In your mind you are the winner, and you feel like a winner. You use every micron of these thoughts, feelings, and emotions to drive you forward to success. No matter what your task is, how challenging or seemingly unreachable your goal, visualisation can help you smash it!

Visualisation is a technique used every day by the world's top performers. Business executives, fighter pilots, surgeons, entrepreneurs, athletes, footballers, gymnasts, sprinters, rowers, martial artists, the lot. It works for people at every level, driving them on to achieve more, pushing their boundaries to excel, be faster, stronger, more dynamic, to reach their goals. It works for them, and it can work for you too.

Military personnel are taught this technique to help them excel on the battlefield and cope should they be captured by the enemy with hardship and potentially torture waiting for them. They are trained to visualise their release from capture. The feeling of being free again, the smell of clean air and freed limbs. The joy of meeting loved ones again. What they will look like, what they will say and do, what they will eat for that first meal, what it will taste like, what drink they will have, what the family chatter around the table will be. The feelings of freedom, the thought of success, the instinct for survival. Right there, powering them on to never give up. There are many accounts recorded by prisoners of war from all the major conflicts paying testament to the value of visualisation and the role it played in keeping them mentally strong.

> Forces beyond your control can take away everything you possess except one thing, your freedom to choose how you will respond to the situation.
>
> - Victor Frankl *Man's Search for Meaning*

How can this technique be used practically in day-to-day life?

Interviews – These can be nerve-wracking, and I admit, even as an experienced police interviewer, I still get nervous when I get interviewed, always have, probably always will. A bit of nerves is good. It keeps you focused, sharp, less likely to make silly mistakes. Nerves are going to be used to our advantage today because they are going to keep us 'on point'.

No matter what interview you go for, it is a reasonable expectation that you've done your preparation and homework (I hope). You've done your research on the job and company, had a look at their website to see what's topical and read up on it. You've completed any paperwork in good time, sought advice from trusted advisers (somebody who works there?), had a scan on social media to see what juicy bits of information might give you the edge over other candidates.

Chef T

A friend of mine was invited for interview for a prestigious role within a famous chain of hotels. He had the letter inviting him in for interview signed by a senior manager, who, it transpired, would be interviewing him. A quick check on her Twitter account revealed her apparent dislike of men with stubble (the thread was about a famous judge on the *X Factor* television programme.) My friend arrived for his interview clean shaven, which is not how he normally presents. Did the fact he was clean shaven contribute to him getting the job? Who knows? Did the fact that he attended clean shaven give him an added layer of confidence that he'd prepared as well as he could? You bet it did!

It doesn't matter how you get the advantage, does it! (As long as it's honest.)

Interviews have a nasty habit of chipping away at your confidence, which in turn drains your resilience. Like anything, prepare as well as you possibly can and sweat the small stuff; it will serve you well.

Back to the interview and here is how visualising success might look. You play this over and over in your mind. You feel every bit of it, every single little piece until you almost hypnotise yourself into it.

You've done your prep. You're ready, happy with your nerves, they're natural. You planned how you're going to get there so arrive in good time. No need to panic. You're sitting in the holding area waiting to be called. Check the facts in your mind. You're ready. You're prepared. You are the right person for this job. You've worked hard to get here, and nothing is going to stand in your way. You are going to go in and deliver your best shot. You are not going to be cocky or complacent. You are going to deliver the best version of you. You are going to smash it.

As the interview concludes, you're going to leave the interview panel with only one choice for the job. You. You are going to remain composed throughout and polite and courteous as you leave. The interview has gone well. You thank the panel for their time and leave the room knowing you have done absolutely everything in your power to deliver. Well done!. Job done. The letter of congratulation is going to look and feel fantastic.

This is just a snapshot of what you might choose to help you grasp the idea. It can work for you in hundreds of settings. Meeting someone for the first time, an exam, speaking in public, a one-to-one with the boss.

I was asked to provide a motivational speech for a team of British canoeists heading out to Canada to compete in the Yukon 1000 challenge. The Yukon 1000 takes you 1000 miles from Canada to the Arctic Circle on an expedition widely recognised as the toughest canoeing challenge in the world. They wanted advice to help them get over the 'wall', the point where they feel exhausted, fed up, drained, and unable to continue during a challenge which pushes your body and soul to the brink. The number-one tip which helped them achieve their goal and finish the race was visualisation. I helped them to 'see' success as they crossed the winning line with friends and family lining the banks of the river cheering them on! I helped them 'feel' the emotion of that moment to give them strength. A simple technique, used many times during the trip, pushing them to go another mile or stay in the water another hour, pushing, encouraging, giving that last bit of 'extra' to push them on to achieve their goals.

- Visualisation activates your creative subconscious which will start generating creative ideas to help you achieve your goal
- It programmes your brain to perceive and recognise the resources you could use to achieve your dreams more readily
- It builds your internal motivation to take the necessary actions to achieve your goals

The cookie jar

It is often said that the best ideas are the simplest. This is one of them. Nothing new here with the science behind the 'cookie jar'. The technique has been taught (perhaps not with this title) and used by military personnel for decades to help prisoners of war survive capture, hardship, and torture. It's all about the mind, what you think, and how you can, in an instant, direct your thoughts to a memory, time, or experience which was positive for you and, in doing so, provide an immediate boost of feel good to 'get you through'.

David Goggins, a retired American marine and ultramarathon runner, captures it perfectly in his book *Can't Hurt Me*, in which he talks about being able to tap into his mental strength reserves to get him through marine training, actually, not just get through, but excel as the team leader. He smashed the course despite being backclassed because of broken legs. Becoming an American special forces soldier is no mean feat in itself, but then he goes on to push himself further, physically and mentally, by taking on some of the world's toughest marathons, including the Badwater Ultramarathon, the 135-mile road race through Death Valley in California. An inferno of blazing, unforgiving July heat. Goggins talks about 'hitting the wall', a term familiar to athletes: the point where you think you've gone as far as you can go, you think that your energy is spent, your lungs are bursting, and your legs are seizing up. You think you can't go any further, the point where you need to find something to push you on and keep you going.

Goggins believes that at this point in the marathon, when you hit the wall, you are only actually about 40 per cent done, there's another 60 per cent left in the tank. He cites the cookie jar as one of the best techniques he knows to help him get over the wall and keep going. It works for him. It works for me. It will work for you. Here's how it works.

You start now. Think about your best memories and moments in your life which gave you your greatest joy. You capture them and put them in your cookie jar, a metaphorical place in your mind where you store all your good memories. When you need or choose to, you dip in and take a cookie, a good memory, an instant boost of energy to push you on.

To give you an idea, I'll share some of mine with you. One of my happiest childhood memories is rock climbing with my friend Paul in the beautiful English Lake District. Happy, carefree days in stunning surroundings. It rains a lot there. We used to camp at the Great Langdale campsite at the head of the Langdale valley. Beautiful, peaceful, but wet! My memory of the sound of the rain on the tent still mesmerises me when I think about it. It's hypnotic. It immediately relaxes me and transports me back to those carefree days. A fantastic memory. Your cookies don't have to be big things either, think special moments. I can still recall my first ever holiday abroad, to Cyprus, walking into the Mediterranean Sea in August for the first time and feeling how warm it was! That first time, the warmth of the water, the heat of the sun on my bones, the sounds of laughter on the beach, the feeling of being completely relaxed and happy. That feeling, that's the point.

The birth of my daughters, getting the letter of acceptance to join the police, meeting my first police dog for the first time, and the sense of achievement I got giving up smoking (I get a lift every January when I see the stop smoking adverts come on the television). Passing my promotion exams and seeing every single one of my daughters' successes as they grow and achieve. Moments which lift me. All cookies. All in my jar.

Your jar can be as big as you want. Fill it! Only recently I happened upon a new cookie by chance. I'm in a supermarket at the self-service checkout, scanning my stuff. In front of me is the walkway leading to the exit. A young mum with a baby girl, dressed in pink in a pram, probably about twelve months old is stopped in front of me, two metres or so from where I'm scanning. I have a perfect view. The mum is talking to a carer pushing an old lady in her wheelchair. She's frail, slow in her movements with a tartan blanket over her to keep her warm. I would say 90 years plus. The push chair and wheelchair are side by side, in touching distance, the women chatting to each other, oblivious to what happens next. The baby turns to the old lady and smiles.

The old lady turns and looks at the baby who holds her hand out towards the lady. Slowly, but deliberately, the old lady inches her tiny frail arm out from under the blanket and reaches towards the baby. They hold hands. The mum and carer carry on chatting. I am captured in the moment. The baby smiles. The old lady smiles. A moment captured forever, a baby bringing a moment of joy to an old lady. They look at each other and then are gone, both women rejoining the hustle and bustle of shopping and the chores of the day. I will never forget that moment. Just like that, right in front of me, new life reaching out to put a smile on the face of a lady moving nearer to the end of hers. That smile. What did it mean to the old lady? It was an incredible moment. I tell this story a lot. My voice always cracks when I do. Very emotional but still lifts me when I think of it.

If you're struggling to think of any cookies to fill your jar, I suggest keeping a journal for a couple of weeks to note them down as they pop into your head, You will have loads, and as you think about it over time, you will be amazed what pops back into your head that you'd forgotten about.

The cookie jar is something you can continue to fill by watching out for those incredible moments which surround us every day. Happy moments, beautiful sights, special, incredible, stand-out moments. Get them in your jar!

Now of course, I'm not suggesting that this technique will turn you into an ultramarathon running special forces soldier! What I am saying is that this is a very powerful technique to know and practise so that if and when you need a lift, if things are not going according to plan, or just because you fancy a treat, you can help yourself to a cookie.

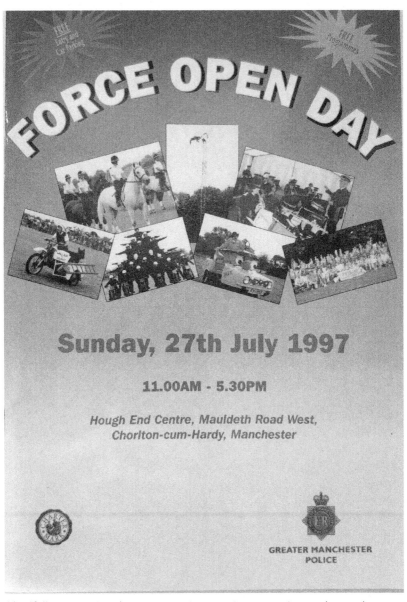

FORCE OPEN DAY

Sunday, 27th July 1997

11.00AM - 5.30PM

*Hough End Centre, Mauldeth Road West,
Chorlton-cum-Hardy, Manchester*

GREATER MANCHESTER
POLICE

Mindfully tapping into happy memories can give you an instant boost. A proven method to stay strong during life's toughest times.

Be mindful

Mindfulness is about being calm and keeping your thoughts fully present in that exact moment in time. How many times have you set off from the house and had to turn back and check whether you locked the door, or driven to work and can't remember the journey? It's because your mind wanders; sometimes that's healthy, sometimes it's not. A mind that wanders will steal your enjoyment of the present moment. The past has gone, don't worry about it. The future isn't here yet, don't worry about it. Being fully present in the moment has numerous benefits. It concentrates your mind. You're able to fully appreciate what's right in front of you. You live your best life. It prevents overthinking and catastrophising. Worrying about loads of different things at the same time can feel like a tsunami, wave after wave hitting you one after the other until you become overwhelmed and drown. During times of increased stress, these waves can feel even bigger and stronger, and if you can't control what's going on, it doesn't take much to completely overwhelm you.

If you'd said to me back in 1989 that one day, as a police officer, I'd be enrolled on a mindfulness course as part of my wellbeing coaching role, I'd have said you were bonkers! Just typing the words, I'm imagining what my colleagues would have said if I'd waltzed into the refs room (police-speak for refreshments room) and started extolling the virtues of being 'mindful', living in the moment and breathing exercises! The culture at the time certainly wasn't ready for that and I would most definitely have received some very direct and to-the-point comments and not very complimentary ones at that! Things were quite different in 2011. A forward-thinking assistant chief constable was leading a revolution in officer wellbeing. A strategic wellbeing board had been set up and I was on it. Greater Manchester Police were a force open to new ideas and willing to try techniques never used before in the police service.

Despite all this positivity around wellbeing and the fact that officer wellbeing was part of my DNA – I lived and breathed it – I must admit I was very sceptical as I entered the classroom on day one of my eight-week mindfulness course. This was for the flower power brigade and people who did yoga. Not for me, a street warrior working the mean streets of Manchester! I was open-minded though and willing to give it a go. My first few lessons didn't go entirely to plan. An early demonstration of breathing techniques saw the whole class lying on yoga mats, fixed on the hypnotic tones of the instructor as she took us through the exercises. It wasn't long before the sound of people breathing, with the occasional fidget, took second place to the noise of quiet snoring as more than a few nodded off on the mats. We were assured that it was normal for beginners learning mindfulness to 'drop off' like this, although those who did were gently but firmly encouraged not to fall asleep again in her class! I know I shouldn't have, but I found it funny. I kept my mirth to myself. The instructor, a softly spoken lady from

Scotland, was so chilled out even a group of hardened street cops weren't going to phase her. Maybe, I thought, if she can stay calm and put up with us lot, there's something in this mindfulness.

The course was excellent. We all got our certificates and a book to further our education into the world of mindfulness. I started to make it part of my daily practice and learn more. I learned that mindfulness is an ancient art form, grounded in the religions of Buddhism and Hinduism and has been around for thousands of years. 'Must be something good about it if it's been going that long,' I thought. I learned how some of the world's leading doctors were using it to treat patients for a whole range of ailments, including pain control, rather than just dishing out tablets. I learned how women use it during childbirth. I learned how the top surgeons use it during surgery to stay calm, rational, and focused. I learned how special forces soldiers use it to stay calm in combat, how snipers use it to control their weapons and shoot accurately, how elite sportsmen and women were able to excel and push themselves even harder just by harnessing the power of breath. I learned how the Royal Navy's top test pilots use it whilst pushing multi-million-pound prototype fighter jets to their limits, and hostage and crisis negotiators stayed cool, calm, collected, and focused to encourage the person not to jump, and at the heart of all this is how you control your breathing. That's enough. I'm convinced. How can I make it work for me?

Take a breather

All the tips, tools and techniques in this book, particularly the breathing stuff is easy to learn and simple to do. So simple in fact, that once you've got the hang of them and start to use them regularly, they become an automatic positive and healthy response to whatever situation you're facing. I call it a 'flinch' response. Imagine a tennis ball flying towards your face. You don't think about blinking or moving quickly to one side to avoid the ball hitting you, if you did pause to think, it would be too late, you'd be hit! Your eyelids automatically close to protect your eyes, your body moves without you consciously thinking about it to avoid the ball crashing into you causing injury. Your brain has taken over and delivered a flinch response, making you blink, and making you move for your protection. That's what we're working towards here with these breathing techniques.

Learning to control your breathing, practising and doing it often enough so that it becomes a flinch response for you is the goal, to reduce stress, anxiety, worry and depression. Used consistently, this technique has the potential to significantly improve your quality of your life and the quality of life for people you care about. And, because our own breathing is a constant resource available to tap into immediately, it can deliver immediate benefits.

Rescue breaths

Three, deep, slow breaths can be enough to create enough time for you to reset and think logically, helping you respond well rather than react badly to whatever's going on immediately in front of you. This technique is probably the simplest and most useful in the whole book. Three big deep breaths will slow your body (your physiology), calm your mind and give you just the right amount of time to think of consequences, actions, and what to do next for the best.

Repeat as many times as you need to until you get the result you want. It is that simple.

You can see in just a few short paragraphs how useful this can be in all our lives and is something you can use immediately. You must keep practising though, I can't stress this enough; we are trying to achieve that flinch response. So, the next time you get into an argument, the delivery guy delivered korma instead of Balti or something else stresses you out, it will kick in and get you through.

Box breathing: the 4-4-4 technique

Box breathing is helpful anytime and particularly during moments of extreme stress. Practise the following process. Inhale for a count of four seconds (some find it easier to time this by actually counting out one thousand, two thousand, three thousand, four thousand) hold your breath in for a count of four seconds, then slowly exhale for a count of four seconds. Wait at the very end of the exhale (all your breath out) for a count of four seconds and repeat the cycle again by breathing in again for a count of four. Repeat as often as you need to. This is a deep breathing exercise that has been shown to calm and regulate the autonomic nervous system. Slowing your breathing in this way allows carbon dioxide to build up in the blood, which stimulates the response of the vagus nerve to produce feelings of calmness throughout the body. (Similar to the effect of breathing into a paper bag for anxious people hyperventilating or having a panic attack.) If you have asthma, COPD, or other similar breathing restrictive conditions, you can adapt the timings to suit your condition, and don't be afraid to consult your physician for further advice.

This is an excellent exercise to get used to the concept of slowing your breathing. Practise at your desk, in your house, whilst driving, doing an exam, going on a date, digging the garden, or brushing your teeth. Practise whilst you're calm, angry or in between, watching TV or eating your dinner, indoors, outdoors up a tree or getting in a lift, it doesn't matter when and where you do it (no one else knows you're doing it!). Have a go and don't be afraid to experiment, tweak the timings and play around to see what works best for you. All I ask is that you practise, practise, practise.

For sleep

Slowing your breathing will calm your mind and body to help you get good quality sleep. A technique I share with police officers who struggle to sleep is the 4-7-8 technique, which involves breathing in through your nose for a count of four seconds, holding your breath for seven seconds, then slow breathing out through your mouth for a count of eight seconds. Repeat until you drift off to sleep. This technique works by calming your body and forcing your mind to concentrate on your breathing rather than the stuff whirring around in your mind. Practitioners report the best results from this one come from regular practice, so it gets better with time, and if you link this with two tips from the sleep section you're onto a winner with the power of three. Again, you can adapt the technique to suit you and try out different variations to see what works best. The internet is also a vast resource for breathing exercises and is well worth a look to see what else is out there which might also serve you well.

The emergency drive

We teach breathing techniques to our police officers to help them stay calm in the most stressful situations.

Imagine you're a police officer receiving an emergency 999 call to a house six miles away from your location. A man is going berserk inside; a woman and two children are barricaded in a room upstairs.

Immediately your heart rate starts to increase and adrenalin kicks in. Got to get there fast!

You get in your police car. Blue lights are on and sirens blaring. It's a long journey at the best of times with 'blues and twos', but it's five o'clock on a Friday evening and the roads around Manchester are busy with tired city centre workers trying to get home to start their weekend.

It is a hazardous, high speed, knuckle-whitening journey to the house. High risk and fraught with danger. Other motorists, tired at the end of the day, careering left and right ahead of you as they inch forward into any space to keep them moving forward. Cyclists with headphones plugged in, unaware of your mission, don't hear you coming and turn right in front of you. Children playing on the pavements, overjoyed it's Friday and no more school, wrapped up in their world of play and totally oblivious to the speeding police vehicle heading right towards them. The young mum with a pram, rushing to cross the road from behind a parked car, more focused on why her baby is crying than what's approaching from her right as she steps out. The man with a white stick and lovely golden retriever...

You are the police driver. It is your responsibility to keep everyone safe. You're highly trained to deal with all of this. The expected and the unexpected. I have to say, police driver training is 'top notch': professional and extremely rewarding to do with some of the most enjoyable courses I ever did in the police, especially the off-road, four-wheel drive course. You get to drive in quarries, through rivers and fields and get paid for it! Really good fun and skills I still use today (albeit not so much driving through rivers anymore!). Anyway back to the emergency.

If you are controlling your breathing, you will be calmer, more focused, and more likely to respond well to the hazards in front of you. You will have a safer, more relaxed drive to arrive at the incident in good order.

You arrive at the address, first at the scene. Three deep slow rescue breaths. You switch off the ignition and exit your car. You move towards the front door, heart rate in check and breathing controlled (flinch response has kicked in throughout the whole drive) allowing you to think rationally. What information do I have about the incident? What do I need? What are my senses telling me? The drive has not phased you; you're calm, focused and ready to deal with whatever's waiting for you behind that door.

Sunrise

A couple of examples demonstrate the benefits. I entered the police station at six in the morning at the start of a beautiful summer's day. We were on earlies, a start at 7 a.m., so we get in early to take a handover from the night team. As I was driving into work, I was mindful (there it is) of a stunning sunrise. A beautiful orange dawn as the sun came up casting a fantastic array of colours across the sky as far as the eye could see. I took it in, fully. A beautiful, short-lived, mindful start to my day which gave me an immediate lift and a great boost I walk to my desk and speak to my sergeants, asking if they'd seen the stunning welcome for us provided by nature as they travelled in. Not one had noticed it. Every one of them engrossed, in their minds, about the workload waiting for them. What they didn't get done yesterday, what will be waiting for them once they get in and what their plans for the day would be. They missed the opportunity.

Nudges

Nudges or baby steps link closely to all the Safe and Sound tips, tools, and techniques and it's another simple tip to use yourself or share with others. When times are tough, workloads excessive or something else is going on in your life which is challenging or stressing you out. Get back to basics and keep things simple. Do something, however small, in the knowledge that you are moving forward. For readers in a management, leadership or coaching role, talking to people about 'baby steps' has a calming effect. It moves people's thinking from an emotional state, perhaps because they feel overwhelmed, back to a logical thinking state in a very quick and easy way, helping to calm them and to see the way forward and light at the end of the tunnel.

When you're going through hell, keep going.

Winston Churchill

I remember being taught a poignant lesson by a mental health crisis support professional who said she always encouraged people in crisis to make their bed when they get up in the morning. By doing this, they've already achieved something (a baby step) in the day, and if the rest of the day goes badly, they will at least have a neat, comfortable, ready-made bed to go to sleep in to get a good night's sleep and try again tomorrow.

Another advantage of using this simple technique is it helps put the brakes on the culture of multitasking, a term and work ethic in fashion for quite a few years which often left people feeling stressed and burnt out. Personally, I've never been a big fan of multitasking for that reason. I've seen many police officers and support staff members succumb to stress because of this concept of being able to spin loads of plates, continually take on more and more in an attempt to do … what? Impress their boss? Peers? Why did they do it? It certainly wasn't good for their health and ruined many people's careers and happiness.

There are exceptions to this of course. In the police, because of the nature of the work and operational necessity, sometimes multiple tasks are considered and actioned together. I'm thinking about firearms incidents, public disorder, or threats-to-life scenarios, but these don't happen all day, every day and, therefore, it means we don't have to, and shouldn't, operate permanently in a multitasking theatre of high stress. One thing at a time, no overthinking, baby steps, sure and steady wins the race.

- Baby steps raise the odds of finishing the task.
- Baby steps are one of most powerful workplace motivators because they are manageable.
- Baby steps promote consistency: key to forming good habits and breaking bad ones.

The next time you're feeling completely overwhelmed, stop. One thing at a time, first things first, start with what is immediately in front of you. Your first step.

Gratitude

Gratitude will help you feel more positive emotions, relish good experiences, improve your health, deal with adversity, and build strong relationships. Gratitude is a powerhouse when it comes to building unshakeable resilience and strong mental health.

From an early age, because of the death of my mum, I had a head start. A life-changing event which showed me how quickly everything can change in an instant. An early lesson in life which helped me develop a 'gratitude' mindset. To appreciate life and all it has to offer fully (mindfulness!). To live life to the full, to seize the day – *carpe diem* – the mantra of many motivational speakers.

Up to now, I think I've achieved that. When my time comes and I'm chosen to meet my maker, I will look back on a full life, well lived, where I appreciated everything life gave me.

Although my life story dictated and crafted this mindset, it was reinforced during studies about wellbeing and resilience. I saw the science behind the way I lived and what I thought brought into focus one Friday evening as my search team and I headed into the city centre of Manchester. Our task, to search the Midland Hotel, an iconic Victorian hotel set right in the heart of the city, famous for the first meeting between Charles Rolls and Henry Royce who would go on to be the founders of Rolls Royce.

We were on an overnight search prior to a royal visit the following day. Our job, to work alongside military search specialists to make sure the hotel and vicinity were safe. No bombs, guns, or other contraband hidden to cause harm or embarrassment during the visit. Our core role as a search team.

As we made our way along Deansgate, the main road which goes right through the city centre, thousands of city-centre workers were making their way home to start their weekend. One of my team moaned in the back of the van: 'I wish I was going home now!'

This negative comment (it was the tone of voice you know) prompted an immediate reply from me.

'How many of the people outside this van right now would give anything to be sat where you are? Police officers, together, doing an important, exciting job tonight rather than sat in front of their computer screens in a boring office job all week counting down the hours to the weekend.' (And before you write in to tell me, I appreciate that not all office jobs are boring.)

A generalisation? Yes. An unfair comparison? Perhaps. Gratitude for the job I do, the opportunity to serve and do exciting work which has meaning, on a task which is important, alongside people I like and respect, in a city I love? Definitely. Gratitude for my lot in the moment and less than one minute to change the perspective of everyone in the van in a positive way which galvanised their resilience and motivation to do a good job that night.

I've asked people to write down a list of everything they're grateful for. Keep it going for a few days and add to the list as things pop into your head. You'll be surprised how much there is and lots you will have forgotten. A list like this can be useful to keep, add to and refer to if you need to.

I did lots of coaching work for a charity in Manchester supporting vulnerable women. Women who had come from the 'school of hard knocks'. Women who'd perhaps had a tough start to life, had been in prison, had, or were having, addiction issues or challenges with domestic abuse. During one of my sessions on gratitude, one woman interrupted me when I started talking about making lists of things I was grateful for. She went on to say that every day, for each of her three children she wrote down one thing on a Post-it note that she was grateful for. They were seemingly small things: good manners, going to bed on time, helping with the household chores, that kind of thing.

On Friday night, she stuck all the Post-it notes up on the wall and showed her children all the things they'd done that week which were good, positive, and mum was grateful for. The children got their chocolate!

Well, I don't know about you, but in my book that counts as outstanding parenting from a mum who only minutes earlier described herself as a 'failure' at parenting. I think not, and she, quite rightly, got a round of applause from the other women in the group. I often wonder how many other women that day went on to do the same thing for their children, a brilliant example of gratitude and how networks can support.

'Are you a glass half full or glass half empty person? Me? I'm just grateful to have a glass'

- Charlie Mackesy – *The Boy, the Mole, the Fox and the Horse*

I encourage you to think about all the things in your life, past and present, that you're grateful for and lean on them at every opportunity for the reasons outlined in the first paragraph above.

Mindfulness, focusing on the present moment, can also help us value and magnify moments and memories of gratitude.

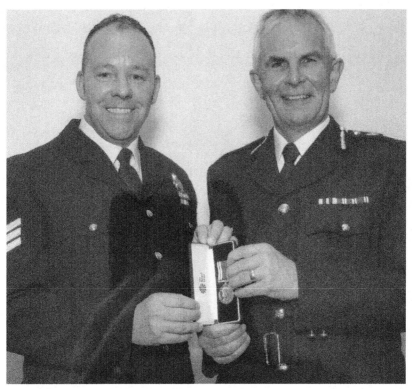

Receiving my Long Service and Good Conduct Medal from the Chief. Grateful to have been given the opportunity to serve.

Catterick

My search team and I were required to relicense once every three years. We would travel as team up to Catterick army camp in the stunningly beautiful county of North Yorkshire where we had to perform numerous search tests under the watchful eye of bomb disposal operators.

The course was generally three days long and, as well as the tests, was a fantastic opportunity to hone our skills and learn from soldiers with experience in bomb disposal and search techniques from Iraq, Afghanistan, Northern Ireland, and other places around the world.

The final day was the exam. It was a pass or fail. Come up to standard or go home unlicensed. The effort we'd all put in had paid off and we all passed. Showered, changed, and out into the lovely market town of Richmond to celebrate. One huge curry and several drinks later, we were in a minibus back to camp. Still buoyed by our success, we had no desire to turn in early and were invited to have drink with the men and women who had instructed on our course. An honour to be invited to drink with real heroes.

The bar was basic but functional, as you would expect from the armed forces. No beer pumps in sight. Cans of lager or Guinness drunk out of the can and a small selection of shorts – vodka or rum. Our night continued.

Spirits were high (excuse the pun) as we laughed, bantered, swapped stories, and made merry. The bar was about half full I'd say, thirty to forty army bods, many still in green camouflage kit having just finished whatever duties they'd been assigned to that day. 'Your round, Russ, get to the bar!'

I manage to stand up (I like rum a bit too much) and move towards the bar, thinking quietly to myself that I'd had enough to drink, and it was time for bed, but it was my round so I get to the bar and stand next to a squaddie in line to be served.

It must have been immediately apparent to him that I wasn't a military man. He enquired, politely, if I was police, with a big grin on his face. I said I was and laughed as he bantered back saying he couldn't believe they let the police in here!

It was good humoured, and he was interested to hear why we were there, and we chatted. And then it happened. A moment which will live me forever. He'd been standing to my left, so I hadn't seen it at first, but as he turned his body towards me I saw that his left arm, at least from the elbow down, was robotic and he had a black metal claw for a hand. This guy had received horrendous injuries in Afghanistan when a roadside bomb detonated, severely injuring him and killing two of his mates.

I sobered up in an instant and my face must have posted a look of horror. He saw me looking and a broad smile lit up his face.

'Go on then, ask me; what do you want to know?' he asked. 'Come on, don't be shy, your mother wasn't!' (He didn't know about my mum, of course.)

We talked for ages. A true hero who laughed in the face of adversity. A man I will never forget. Courageous, heroic, resilient. A man who found it cathartic to talk about what had happened. An amazing ambassador for our armed forces and the men and women who serve.

I can only imagine what he's been through. What I can say, though, is this: I will always respect our military personnel for what they do, and I will never, ever, take my hands for granted ever again.

CHAPTER 3

Humour

Laughter can take the heat out of most situations. It's like the valve on the top of the pressure cooker opening to let steam out. Humour cools things down. The designers of Blackpool's Pleasure Beach theme park knew this over a hundred years ago when they put a huge laughing clown at the entrance to greet visitors as they arrived. They knew that the sight and sound of the clown's laughter would make people laugh, reduce stress and set the tone for a great day out for the mill workers of Lancashire as they flocked to the seaside resort for some fun and respite away from the dangers and long hours working in the cotton mills.

Finding humour and having a good laugh has been a tool for wellbeing which has endured through the ages.

Manchester looters

I was involved in two major bomb incidents during my career with Greater Manchester Police. The first was on 15 June 1996. The IRA had parked a lorry packed with explosives at the side of the Arndale Centre, a huge multi-floor shopping complex packed with shoppers in the heart of the city centre. Thankfully, the terrorists also provided security services with a codeword to afford time to evacuate this huge city, and because of that and the speedy response by emergency teams to get everyone out, no one was killed or seriously injured.

The memories which surface when I think back to that day are the ones which make me smile now, just as they did back then. Memories of the six women sitting under hair dryers having their hair blow-dried in a high-class coiffeur on Deansgate. Asked to leave by police officers because of the impending explosion, they replied with: 'Can we have another 30 minutes to finish off?' Funny? It shouldn't be, when you're trying to evacuate thousands of people and secure a massive area, but it was. A moment of mirth to let out a bit of pressure in a stressful day, it kept us going. I'm pleased to say the ladies came round to our way of thinking and grudgingly left the hairdressers, albeit looking a bit windswept! They survived to be cut and blown again.

The biggest bomb to be detonated in the UK since World War II caused widespread devastation. The only thing in the area untouched by the blast was the red post box on Corporation St. which stood strong. A photograph flashed around the world and is used to this day to represent the resilience of Manchester and its people. The post box remains in the same spot today, a small plaque added as a reminder for those who care to stop and read.

A cordon is placed around the city centre. Everybody's out. A huge crime scene which, in the coming days, will be examined, pored over, searched, and photographed. But for now, we are one of three serials (a sergeant and six constables on each) patrolling inside the cordon in an armoured personnel carrier.

It's a deserted city. A surreal, apocalyptic experience. I will never forget the silence in an area I knew well. Silent except for the sound of glass crunching and grinding under our wheels as we crawled along at walking pace, the occasional smash of shattered windows falling to the ground from office blocks high above us, splintering into a million razors on the ground. The relentless chatter of window blinds rattling in the breeze from a thousand broken windows.

We move slowly through the streets taking in the macabre sights unfolding around us at every turn. Up Market St. toward Debenhams department store, every one of the huge display windows blown out. The voids within reveal the shadowy form of two females clambering out of the shop through the mess of mannequins which was once a neat display of high-class clothing. Both were dressed for the occasion. Low cut blouses, miniskirts, and high-heeled shoes. Exactly the right attire for a bomb site shopping spree! Each had two large bags with them, crammed to the brim with stolen cosmetics. They were looters and the only two people on Market St. at that time … apart from us!

They walk towards us, smiling. They know the game is up. The carrier stops.

'Do you know the way to the bus station love?' The tallest one asks, still smiling and holding her bags as if this was just another normal day out.

'It's closed at the moment, no buses running through the city centre,' replies the sergeant, smiling back from his front-row seat.

'Trains?' she continues.

No trains either at the moment. Have you got far to go?'

'Salford, love! Any chance of a lift?' She sounds upbeat and hopeful.

They know they won't be going home any time soon and probably regretted choosing stilettos over trainers. At least a decent pair would have given them a chance to make a run for it, but no, not in six-inchers.

'Jump in, we're heading your way as it happens. Via Pendleton Police Station. You're both under arrest for theft.' Everybody is still smiling. It's weird.

Humour can be found in the darkest of places and the most unlikely situations. People say that emergency service workers, police, fire, ambulance, nurses, and the military develop a warped sense of humour. It's true. It releases the pressure and helps you cope. It gets you through and it doesn't have to be the big events, it's humour in everyday moments which are gold.

The two officers who 'linked' each arm of a 25-stone woman and sang Frank Sinatra's famous song 'New York, New York' and high-kicked their way into North Manchester Accident and Emergency department on a busy Friday night. A tactical method not found in any mental health awareness book anywhere in the world. It worked. It got her in for treatment (much to the amusement of the doctors and nurses waiting to receive her and the drunks sitting in the waiting room).

The new police officer handcuffed to a kettle and left there until he agreed to brew up for the team. His ego tamed because he thought brewing up was 'beneath him'.

An officer on the team being pushed around the station on a wheeled office chair because he 'needed to speed up' having just failed to catch a fleeing criminal during a foot chase.

The dog handler who thought it would be a good idea to tie his German Shepherd's leash to the bumper of his car whilst he groomed the dog. The dog pulled the bumper off the car and ran off down the street with it clanging behind him, dog on one end of the leash, bumper on the other.

Officers' nick names also provide a light moment...

Splash – Arrested a thief in a stolen car but failed to put the handbrake on and watched in dismay as it rolled down the hill into a pond.

Mesmo (the memory man) – Overslept numerous times because he 'forgot' he was on the early shift. The nickname stayed with him and is still with him in retirement.

Blank – The expression on an officer's face every time the sergeant asked for her paperwork which was overdue (again).

In times of war

Finally, in honour of our military personnel, a brief visit to the trenches during WWI. Scene of unimaginable horror, suffering and death. Amidst all this, men found ways to laugh, to banter, to keep spirits up so they could continue to fight. This spirit captured by the comedic antics of 'Old Bill' in the Ypres Times, an early comic nicknamed the Wipers Times by the Tommies because it was easier to say! Old Bill would tell jokes and make fun out of everything: the food, the mud, the weather, the cigarettes, the Germans, nothing was excluded. A powerful example of finding something positive out of darkness to keep spirits up.

All these moments are around us every day, even during our toughest times, although sometimes the darkness means we must look harder to find them. Moments to laugh, moments for fun, moments which lift you, galvanise your resilience, drive you on and help you get through and achieve extraordinary things as it does for our front-line emergency responders, our armed forces and all those who thrive during tough times.

My message about humour and the role it plays in building unshakeable personal resilience and strong mental health is this.

Please don't let any opportunity to smile, laugh out loud, and have fun pass you by. Go out of your way to make those moments happen. Cherish them, encourage them, appreciate them, look for them, notice them, and build them into your life.

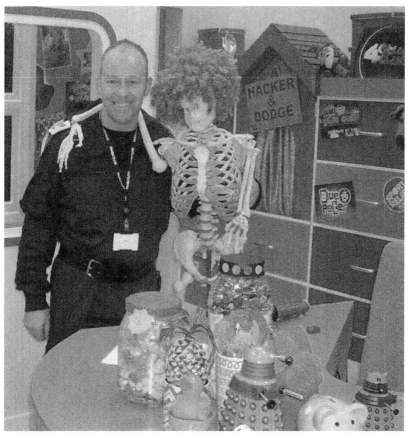

Never let an opportunity to smile pass you by.

Reset

Take a break. A few seconds, minutes, maybe an hour or two. Perhaps it's a week on holiday or longer. Reset is about kindness to yourself, giving yourself a breather to slow down and take stock of things. A word we use a lot in the police is 'decompress'. I like this word a lot: it nails it in one.

Reset is all these things. It starts with awareness of when you need a break – emotional intelligence, if you want to be specific. Maybe someone has given you a clue that you need to reset. You've got a bit tetchy perhaps, said or done something out of character, you feel stressed, and this has manifested itself in your behaviour (well zone to wobble zone).

I have a small red emergency smash button (like you might see on an escalator to stop it in an emergency) to visually demonstrate this during my workshops. The button is not much to look at, nothing fancy, purchased from an electrical gizmo store in Manchester, but its significance and what it stands for can have a huge impact on you and your resilience if you don't press it to reset when you need to, leaving you stressed, burning out, not thinking clearly, making poor decisions and reacting badly to what's in front of you instead of responding well.

Three tips to reset immediately:

- Slow your breathing to slow your mind (you knew this would be here!). Focus on the here and now. This can be done any time, any place anywhere. I'm hoping you are practising now!
- Go outside and breathe in fresh air, be amongst nature if you can. Find green.
- Move your body. Exercise, go for a walk, run, climb stairs if this is your only option right now. Do something to raise your heart rate and pump oxygen around your body. It will energise and refresh you.

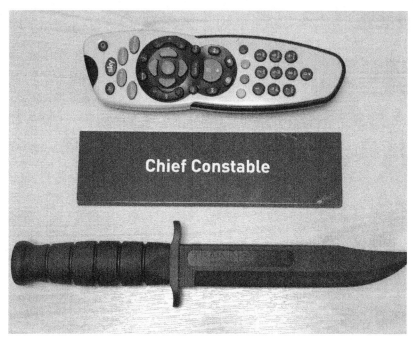

Building and maintaining resilience and mental strength is the number one life skill and is important for everyone, no matter who you are.

Acceptance

Let me get straight to the point. Life can be tough at times. Accepting your feelings for what they are is exactly what it says on the tin. There are people who live in what I believe is a fantasy world, where everything is rosy and sunny and calm. That is not my world. I am a realist and the message I share is encouraging you to become 'comfortable with being uncomfortable'. Accepting your feelings for what they are, grounded in mindful practice, not beating yourself up because you had a bad day, or you feel bad in the moment. Yes, loads of learning can come when things aren't going so well and you feel bad, I'm happy that you dwell on that. What I won't do is flower it all up. Sometimes, to use an Americanism, life sucks.

Here's a selection of incredibly valuable tips, tools, and techniques to help you through.

- By now you have started to build your spokes, you're practising them and seeing what works for you. Let your spokes hold you up.
- Know that feelings come and go, this will not last forever.
- Don't beat yourself up for feeling bad, guilty, upset, disappointed. It's normal, natural, and OK.

You may have heard of the term 'what doesn't kill you makes you stronger'; here's a different perspective on it.

Old Man Wolverine

Old Man Wolverine is a superhero toy I use to demonstrate this technique in my workshops. He's about six inches tall, made of plastic and has a huge muscular torso and massive muscular arms (but stick-thin legs because he 'skipped' leg day!).

He features because of his muscular physique, and I don't have to tell you that big muscles make you stronger. The mind is also a muscle, and I want to make the case that you can build mind muscle in a similar way to the way you build muscles in your body.

Wolverine, like us, needs three things to make the muscles in his body grow.

1. Stress them by lifting heavy weights.
2. Feed them quality protein to nourish them.
3. Rest them so they repair and grow back bigger and stronger than they were before.

You can use the same approach to change your thinking and move your thoughts back to a positive space when things go wrong. Instead of stressing and dwelling on things negatively when somethings have not gone according to plan, think of it this way.

1. You've stepped outside your comfort zone and had a go. You've stressed your mind in a good way by trying new ideas and experiences and that's what life's all about.

2. You've fed your mind with the experience and knowledge about what works and what doesn't.

3. You reflect on what's happened, knowing that no matter what the outcome, you're growing stronger, wiser, and better prepared to go again.

It's always about what you think.
- Author

Old Trafford – We learn most when things go wrong

I spent twelve months as a temporary inspector prior to getting my full promotion. This means you're given the insignia and powers of the full rank yet still have to officially qualify at an assessment centre for full confirmation in the rank. The temporary rank gives you a chance to gather experience and evidence to demonstrate your competence. It's a privileged opportunity.

Barely three months into my new temporary role and I'm given the opportunity to police a football match at Manchester United's Old Trafford football ground. An iconic location in Stretford in the heart of Manchester. I'm not a huge football fan, and my knowledge of football is poor, but I knew United were playing a European side in the Champions League competition. I'd read the intelligence. No threats or crowd trouble expected, very few travelling supporters expected and, in any event, Greater Manchester Police have an excellent reputation for preventing disorder at Old Trafford. I'm very relaxed as we head towards Stretford Police Station in three armoured personnel carriers for the pre-match briefing. I'm sitting, as the inspector (albeit temporary) in the lead vehicle, responsible for a full police support unit: that's me, three sergeants and twenty-one constables, all of whom were my responsibility. I'd been sent the operational order about two weeks prior to the day but I'd been busy with other things, and in the back of my mind, everything would be OK at the match, so I didn't feel the need to read it. This is the booklet that tells you everything you need to know about the game. Information on the teams, who's working where and all the emergency procedures. I knew the ground well having worked there as a sergeant many times and, with there having been no problems, anticipated this would be a breeze.

I wasn't there as a sergeant though, was I?

The pre-match briefing completed, we marched to the ground. The visiting fans were vocal and good natured until they got inside the ground. Almost immediately the whistle blew to start the game, the trouble started. Missiles, including coins and stones, were thrown at United fans and onto the pitch at the players, flares were let off, officers and stewards were under attack. This was not part of the plan.

I was requested by the control room to move my teams in to support, but I didn't know where the right zone to move into was. I hadn't read the booklet. The disorder continued, and at one point, the match was stopped for offenders to be arrested or ejected from the ground and calm to be restored. Whilst all this was going on, I was wandering around feeling lost. Where were my sergeants? They were with their teams in the right zones, directed there by match control, but where was I? Again, I struggled to understand. I hadn't studied the full layout of the ground (as an inspector must) and didn't know where I or my teams needed to be. I fell well short of what was expected of me, and it was only thanks to the professionalism of my sergeants that everything was eventually OK.

Things didn't improve after the game. I can only describe it as chaos. My sergeants and constables did an outstanding job supported by Tactical Aid Units, police horses, police dogs and the other police units in attendance. Every one of my team knew what they were doing. They had prepared properly. The odd one out was me.

The drive home was a quiet affair. Although everyone was polite to me, I knew that they knew that I'd done a rubbish job, and it hurt. A long period of reflection and 'beating myself up' followed. I vowed that I would never ever fail to prepare properly again. Thankfully, none of my officers had been injured on that day, but what if they had and it was because of me? That weighed heavily on my mind for weeks. It still does now.

They say you learn most when things don't go according to plan and that's true. What is vital though, is how you deal with those things, what you think and what you feel. If I'd known the analogy of Old Man Wolverine back then, I would still have learned my lesson, for sure, but I wouldn't have been so hard on myself. I believe that can make a huge difference. Perhaps even the difference between life and death

Fear kills more dreams than failure ever did.

Handcuffs – Be wary of getting locked into negative patterns of thoughts behaviours and language.

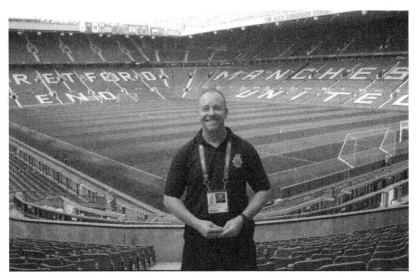

Old Trafford Manchester: An Iconic football ground but not always the theatre of dreams.

A valuable piece of police equipment which has been used by police officers for hundreds of years to restrain people who are violent, likely to injure themselves or others, or try to escape. The design of handcuffs has changed over the years, from the very heavy 'snaps' of the Victorian era through to cuffs joined by a short chain made up of four links right up to the modern-day Kwik Kuff rigid handcuff. A hugely impressive piece of kit with multiple uses.

The 'small chain' version which I was issued with in 1989 could be hard to apply to a detainee's wrists, particularly if they were violent. As soon as the officer got one cuff on the first wrist, the remaining cuff was free to be used as a weapon if it wasn't controlled and applied to the perpetrators second wrist quickly, becoming a flailing steel weapon capable of inflicting horrendous gashes, broken noses and eye injuries to unlucky or unprepared officers.

The modern-day cuffs are solid with no chain. Even the application of one cuff allows the officer a tremendous amount of control. They receive comprehensive training on how to apply reasonable force to perpetrators' wrists to exert control should this be required; this includes 'take downs' and various different handcuffing techniques, all designed to keep the perpetrator restrained yet keep them and the officer safe.

One thing which has never changed is the interest this piece of kit evokes in young people and adults alike. Few people can resist the opportunity to have a go to see what it feels like to play 'cop' or 'robber', and it has been a staple exercise of neighbourhood police officers for years when doing school engagement visits.

The reason I mention handcuffs here is twofold. The first is that resilience, like handcuffing techniques, can be taught (and should have frequent refresher training). The second is a message about getting 'locked in' to negative thoughts and patterns of behaviour which impact negatively on you, your behaviour, and your resilience. Negative self-talk is by far the most common, with some almost hypnotising themselves into believing that 'I'll never be able to'; 'I'm not good enough'; 'I can't'.

Notice when these self-limiting 'beliefs' start to crop up and challenge them. The saying goes that you are what you think, and I've seen many competent, capable people, police officers included, talk themselves out of dream jobs, relationships, promotion and more simply by repeating negative chatter in their mind. Watch for it. Notice it. Challenge it.

I also encourage you to reflect on your own behaviours and choice of language. Does the way you behave or speak cause trouble? Are you able to listen to your partner when they need you to, or do you switch off? How do you respond to criticism? What do you do and say when an unforeseen obstacle gets put in your way or you meet a challenge? How do you act when you're tired and hungry? I don't have to tell you how these little things quickly become big things over time, ruining relationships, eroding happiness, and battering your mental wellbeing. So, encouragement to reflect on the dangers of becoming locked into negative patterns of thinking, behaviour, and language. What positive changes could you make today?

The tough cookies

There will always be the 'tough cookies'. Those individuals who won't or can't talk about how they are. You may be one of them. This can be a defence mechanism: *If I don't talk about it, I won't be opening any painful wounds.* We see this a lot in military personnel. It can be the culture: *This is a tough job, I'm tough, I can cope with anything, I just crack on.* It can be that people are fearful of repercussions: *If I open up to my boss and tell him or her personal things about me, it might be used against me sometime in the future, for promotion perhaps.* (See where trust comes in here?) It can be pride: *Keep it hidden and then I won't be embarrassed about it by talking or telling anyone.* This culture of non-disclosure can be prevalent in industries and organisations where a macho culture exists (such as the police). It also exists in organisations with no psychological safety net in place so that people are safe and, just as importantly, **feel safe** to talk.

If you're reading this now and you recognise yourself, I ask you to consider how well you'd cope if you were suddenly faced with a catastrophic situation in your life: something which comes out of the blue and completely overwhelms you. I am certainly not judging, and there are people who manage perfectly well by not talking, and if that works for you, who am I to preach? What I would ask you to consider though, is what the effect might be on your physical and mental health further down the line if you consistently bottle things up.

I have three questions to help you reflect.

- How do you control your stress?
- How do you decompress?
- Do you have enough 'spokes in your wheel' to lean on now and in the future should you need it, and if not, could you be susceptible to post-traumatic stress later in life?

It is exactly for these reasons that I encourage all blue light emergency services and military personnel to find opportunities to talk openly. By building your resilience early on and engineering strong spokes into your wheel, you will be far better equipped to deal with challenges and bounce back at every point during your journey through life. You will have something to lean on.

Dave and his domestic dilemma

Dave had been a police officer on my team for over two years, and I knew him well. He was what we call 'a good lad'. Experienced, hardworking, reliable, calm in a crisis and perfectly suited to work on the 'van'. The van was generally a Ford Transit or something similar with specialist equipment on board, search stuff, powerful lighting, evidence-gathering paraphernalia, ladders and wham rams (a large metal battering ram for getting into houses quickly) and an armoured cage in the back for transporting prisoners. It was normally crewed by two experienced officers.

The van crew have a critical role to play on the team, responding to pub fights, disputes, calls for back-up, stabbings, and burglaries in progress. They transport prisoners, visit crime scenes, gather evidence, reassure victims of crime and are the first to respond to emergency calls. The van goes to anything and everything and is often seen as the best duty to have, generally given to the more experienced officers on the team.

Dave was a handy lad, able to look after himself when needed and someone you were glad was on your side when the chips were down. He was also a competent communicator, skilled at calming situations and could keep his cool even in the face of extreme provocation. He had the knack of knowing just what to say to settle people who were frightened, calm people who were angry, and stop those who were foolish from talking themselves into the back of the van.

Dave's partner for many months was Kat. An officer of similar calibre. They had a fantastic bond which enabled them to bounce off each other and find humour in almost everything they did – which helped them cope with their lot. They worked well together and could be relied on to handle anything asked of them. A sergeant's dream team.

Dave and Kat knew each other well. Ten hours working together every day meant they got to know a lot about each other: what made each other tick, their strengths and weaknesses, each other's hopes, dreams and desires and everything in between.

Kat was the first to notice Dave's temperament change from calm, cool, professional to short-tempered and irritable – with her and members of the public. She challenged him.

It transpired that Dave and his wife had not been getting on for a while and she'd left him. He still loved her at that time and hadn't wanted the marriage to end, although she saw it very differently. A common scenario in society, but Dave was struggling with it, and this was the underlying issue driving his behaviour. A couple of complaint forms for 'abuse of authority' (being disrespectful to members of the public) landed unexpectedly on my desk. As his boss, it was my job to sort it. It doesn't matter who you are and whether I like you or not, being disrespectful to the public is unacceptable and I will deal with it. The question for me though, was **why**? Kat had already mentioned to me about his wife and had told me in confidence, 'He's a proud man and doesn't want to tell the rest of the team and risk breaking down in front of them.' I understood that and assured Kat I would be discreet.

Dave entered my office and sat down. We talked about the complaints. He admitted he'd been short-tempered and took full responsibility. I was grateful for his honesty. Thankfully, both complainants accepted an apology, and the matter was closed. But what about the future? Was he OK? Dave assured me that there would be no further complaints. I believed him. I asked him if he wanted to talk, explaining that I'd heard about the situation with his wife, I wasn't prying, but was here to support him if needed. He assured me he didn't need or want to talk about it and asked if we were done. As he got up to leave my office, I passed him a bit of paper with my personal phone number on with the offer of a listening ear and a coffee, anytime, on or off duty.

Dave never rang or got any more complaints. He and Kat continued to work well together as a team; she continued to be his rock and my eyes and ears on the ground. I continued to check in with Kat and Dave regularly to make sure all was OK.

'How's things?' I enquired discreetly. 'How is Dave?' and just as importantly, 'How are you?'

Questions grounded in trust and mutual respect and a genuine desire to support and care.

All ended well as it normally does with these things. Very painful at the time with lots of upheaval, financial and emotional stress but, ultimately, when everything settles and with the passage of time, we move on.

There is a fine line to tread being the boss. I care for my team, and I want them to be OK, but I also have a job to do. I have a responsibility to the community we serve, and I have a responsibility to the wider team. I also have a responsibility to deal with poor performance. All these responsibilities require my attention. All are important. Experience, wisdom, and professional judgement are all needed if the delicate balance between all is to be maintained.

Some weeks later, Dave called in to tell me his divorce was complete, and he'd moved on. He appreciated how I'd handled the complaints and apologised for putting me in the position of having to deal with them. One of his strongest spokes was Kat. Dave spoke to her throughout; she was his listening ear in the cab of a Ford Transit at four in the morning when most of the city was asleep. He didn't need me. The bit of paper with my number on was all he needed, just to know he could ring if he needed me was enough. And what about Kat's disclosure about Dave's marriage to me? In some quarters that would have been gossip but not in this situation. The passage of information between people you trust, who have only your best interest at heart, is not gossip. It's the oil which keeps the wheels of wellbeing turning, delivered from an oil can galvanised by love and respect for each other.

As a resilience coach, it's knowing when to step in and when to back off. Knowing who can support you to support others and how they will do this. It's knowing your own limitations and, ultimately, delivering the right approach for each different scenario. Summed up perfectly by Nannie McPhee in the film of the same name.

When you need me but don't want me, I'll be there. When you want me but don't need me, I'll be gone.

We need to talk

Nobody wants to hear those words; what they really mean is 'You're in trouble'!

My take is quite different. If I had to name one thing, one spoke, one top tip, tool, or technique related to strong personal resilience, it's this: IT IS GOOD TO TALK. Capital letters, it must be important, and it is. Let's dig a bit deeper.

The Japanese have a saying. You have three 'faces'. One you show the world, one you show friends and family, and one you show only to yourself. This last one is the one we're interested in now and the one I'm interested in when you sit with me. This third face is the one which represents your deepest thoughts, worries, concerns, and beliefs. The face you show yourself when you're alone, on the bus, in the car, walking the dog, or sitting alone in your bedroom. This is the face you show no one. We all have one.

Andy

Andy was the team clown and made everybody laugh. A fantastic police officer. A big strong lad, popular with everyone and the life and soul of the party. He'd been on the team for over ten years and, on the face of things, seemed to be well adjusted, happy, and well. No one ever expected to hear the news that morning on the seven o'clock parade that Andy had taken his own life. It left us all devastated.

We saw his 'public face'. We never saw the face he showed only to himself. The stuff going on in his mind had overwhelmed him. Andy's death left us all reeling. Why didn't we know? How could we have prevented it? Why didn't he tell us he was struggling? A lot of soul searching for us and his family to try to find a reason, a chink, a sliver of something to help us rationalise what had happened. The truth was, we couldn't have. It was Andy's decision, no matter how upsetting that was for us.

I remember having a conversation with a counsellor from the Samaritans (an online mental health support charity who do a fantastic job supporting people in crisis) shortly after Andy's death. They are trained to speak to people on the brink of suicide and help them find a way back from the edge. I asked him how he coped when someone he'd been supporting, on the phone say, goes on to take their own life. His reply was straight to the point.

'I will help anybody as much as I can, but what I can't do is take away someone's self-determination to take their own life if that's what they want to do.'

His bluntness shocked me. I quietly wondered how we was able to be so matter of about it. It seemed at odds with the caring compassionate service the Samaritans provide. I am not judging, and I'm certainly not criticising; this man was a trained professional and a volunteer, giving his time up to help others for no financial reward. His response was how he rationalised and made sense of the saddest parts of his work. It was a coping mechanism which allowed him to be able to do the job he does.

Suicide takes over 6500 lives in the UK every year: men, women, and children who see suicide as their only way out. Three-quarters of them were men. Shocking isn't it?

If you're struggling right now please remember you're never alone. There are people who love you, care about you and are ready right now to help you. There is always another way out, although sometimes it's hard to see. Talk to someone, go online to seek help or pick up the phone. I promise you'll be glad you did and so will those who love you,

Talking brings light to the darkness and will help you find your way, whether that's the day-to-day challenges we all face or the devastating life-changing catastrophic challenges which seem unsurmountable.

If you've ever been in the position where things are getting too much and stress is overwhelming you, it can feel like a ball of tangled wool in your head. Talking helps to unravel it all. Talking helps to make sense of it by unravelling it all then winding it back up in neat compact bundles of logic and sense.

Keeping things bottled up is not good for you. My favourite analogy is of an acid slowly corroding and burning you from the inside. I want to share with you the case for talking regularly about how you are, what you're thinking and feeling as the number one thing for keeping you going and diluting the acid.

There's nothing new in this either. Our grandparents taught us: *A trouble shared is a trouble halved.*

As true today as it was back then!

Talking gets stuff out. It dilutes the acid and makes it less harmful. Talking gets 'stuff' out and onto the (figurative) table. From there, you can shine a light on it, reduce the darkness, and expose it. Talking helps to unravel the mess, the feelings, the worry, the concerns. Talking helps you to start to make sense of what's going on. Different analogies all used hundreds of times throughout my career during conversations with tough front-line police officers to help them make sense of the madness. It worked for them. It will work for you.

Talking, for some, is hard to do. Who do you talk to? What do you say? What if pride gets in the way or you're too shy? What if you're embarrassed? What if you're the chief executive officer, team leader, or boss and feel there's no one to turn to because of your position? What if you want to talk to your boss but feel it will hinder your career or be used against you by someone with dubious integrity? (All of these are your third face remember.) So many 'what ifs' which become barriers to talking if we let them.

Experience shows that there is likely to be more damage caused by NOT talking than there is by speaking out.

I want to make the case for knowledge. You're increasing this now by reading this book. I encourage you to learn more about talking as a healthy thing to do. I want to make the case for practice. Practise talking so that as you notice yourself moving from the well to wobble zone, it's there, immediately useable as one of your spokes to support you early enough to stop things spiralling out of control: wobble to wipe-out? We are not going there!

I want to encourage you to talk about the benefits of talking. Use my analogies or use your own, use personal stories, it doesn't matter how you do it, there's no exact science with any of this. You take the principle – talking is good for you – and make it your own, you mash it, tweak it, mould it, and communicate it in a way which is your natural communication style. By doing this, you speak from the heart, you are authentic, honest, and trustworthy and people will listen to you. In turn, you will be helping others and that is good for you too.

For those in a position of influence or authority, as soon as you start to talk about 'how you are', you start to create the psychological safety net which give others 'permission' to open up and talk about how they are. A brilliant thing which will enhance the culture of your organisation, strengthen your friendships, make your family bonds even stronger, and set you all on the path to unshakeable resilience and strong mental health.

When you put this book down today and before you go to sleep tonight, ask this question to someone close to you and see where it takes you.

'Why is talking good for your mental health?'

The phones

I had over one hundred one-to-one wellbeing conversations with staff who'd been involved with the Manchester Arena bombing in 2017. Some of those conversations will never leave me.

Rooms were available for anyone to have quiet time, relax, decompress, seek advice, or talk about their experience to 'offload'.

From all these conversations, there's one which stands out for me. It demonstrates perfectly the value of talking.

On the night of the attack, the initial scenes were chaotic whilst the area was made safe. Injured people given first aid and transferred to hospital and police cordons put in place. Once this phase was complete, Manchester City Centre was in lockdown. A quiet, surreal experience with only the sound of occasional sirens in the distance to break the eerie silence across this normally bustling city.

The concourse of the arena had been secured as a crime scene. Blue police tape surrounding it with police officers guarding all entrance and exit points. Nobody going in to prevent vital evidence being disturbed. A scene of horror and devastation where 23 people lost their lives.

The person who walked into my room that morning was a senior detective on duty that night. Tasked with entering the scene with a small group of forensic scientists and a photographer, all covered head to toe in white suits to prevent contamination of evidence.

Their solemn task was to assess the scene and commence the criminal investigation.

He sat down opposite me, invited in because he'd been identified as 'high risk' (as everyone who entered the scene was) and, potentially, in need of specialist welfare support. I'd seen him before, we knew each other to say hello, but that was about it. It was a small room, three chairs, a small round table in the middle, a sink, lamp, and box of tissues on the table.

We exchanged pleasantries.

I explained what my role was, and the different welfare options Greater Manchester Police were providing for staff to support their wellbeing. He sat bolt upright, legs crossed, hands clasped tightly together in his lap. His hands were completely white, almost bloodless it seemed as he was clasping them so tightly. My first clue that all was not well, perhaps?

He looked slightly bemused as he told me that he was OK and went on to say that he knew it was always going to be difficult going into the scene, but he'd been a detective a long time and had seen lots of death and destruction during his career. It was his job and his duty to go in and after all, as a seasoned detective, he'd 'been in hundreds of crime scenes to start the rigid process of murder investigation.' He told me he could cope with it. His hands suggested differently. Clamped together like he was holding onto a rollercoaster. His knuckles were white.

I remained quiet. Most of my work involves being quiet and listening. He carried on talking. I listened. He talked for about twenty minutes about his role, what he did, what he saw, who else was there and his family.

'Are we done now?' he asked. His hands provided the answer.

'Are you sleeping OK?' I asked him (changes to sleep patterns being a good indicator for me). I kept quiet. There was a long silence, probably a minute or so, but it seemed a lot longer. I knew there was something.

'It's the phones,' he said, slowly and quietly, a tear rolling down his cheek.

He looked me directly in the eyes. 'I can't get the sound of the phones out of my mind. I don't sleep because of the phones.'

I felt relief.

The phones he was referring to were the mobile phones owned by and still in the possession of the deceased. Ringing constantly. Families, desperate for them to be answered to hear their loved one's voice and know that they were was safe. It wasn't going to be. Multiple phones, ringing constantly, a haunting sound breaking up the silence as he moved slowly through the concourse and amongst the deceased, formulating his plan.

The thought of this is enough to move anyone to tears. We both cried. The writing of these words now does not in any way do justice, if that's the right word, to the emotion we both felt in that room right then. It was overwhelming, but it was a good thing for him. Cathartic. An emotional release, and he needed that.

There is a point to sharing this sad story and painful memory with you here.

My colleague was able to talk about that bit of the whole experience which was hurting him and keeping him awake at night. The piece of the jigsaw, which was sitting in the corner of his mind, corroding from the inside. He was able to 'get it out of his head'. He told someone. No further dissection or wellbeing support was needed. My colleague left the room. He talked, his trouble shared, his trouble halved. He sleeps well again.

If reading this story has inspired you to think differently about the value of talking, the tears shed whilst writing this will have been worth it, and if you go on to empower and encourage others, the pain, for me, will be less.

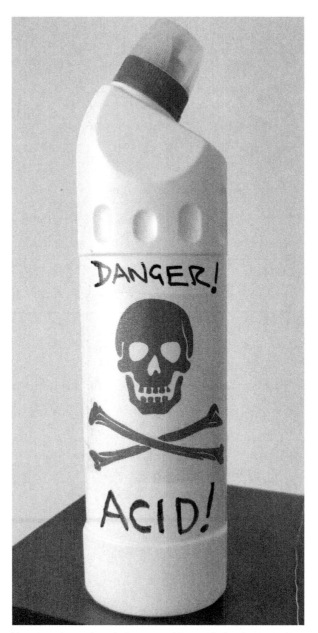

Keeping things bottled up acts like acid slowly corroding from the inside. Talking dilutes the acid. Vital for mental strength.

I'm too busy

'I'm too busy!' 'There's not enough time!' 'I can't believe they're asking me to do this on top of everything else!' 'I've already got too much to do.'

We live in a busy world and it's easy to get 'locked in' to the belief that there isn't enough time to do everything you want or need to do. As the financial crash started to bite in 2008, every police force across the country found itself having to make financial savings with staff numbers the hardest hit. Numbers of front-line police officers were dramatically reduced as were back-office functions. Administration teams, uniform and equipment stores, and prosecution file preparation were three areas which were culled, having a huge impact on front-line police officer's workload and ability to function.

The nature of the job was also changing. National recording standards were introduced by the government, meaning officers were recording more reports of crime. Even a Sunday morning verbal spat between two dads at their sons' football game would have to be recorded as a public order incident, triaged and investigated. Workload rocketed and that's before we add on the threat from online crime, cyber-attacks and the thousands of complaints generated by social media, such as 'Little Johnny' telling 'Little Bob' that he's not his 'best friend forever' anymore.

One of the most bizarre reports I recall was the man who rang the police because his neighbour's apple tree was overhanging his garden!

Supporting staff through change processes was all part of my work as a resilience coach and hardly a day went by without a chat with someone about workload and how to manage it better.

These are a few of the techniques I found useful myself and shared with my teams.

First things first

I know, immediately, that this will sound patronising. I'm sorry about that but please bear with me. We all know that putting first thing first is common sense, but hand on heart, who can say they live by this mantra? One of Steven Covey's rules from his international bestselling effective leadership and management book *The Seven Habits of Highly Effective People*. I read it a few years ago and, like you might be now, felt quite annoyed that this supposedly bestselling book was telling me something as simple as this!

The thing to do is reflect on how you operate. The stuff you do, habitually, that is stealing your time and affecting your performance, health, and happiness. Take social media. Do you pick up your phone and look at it when there is something more important to do? Especially if that something isn't what you particularly want to do? Do you pay more attention to your phone than you do to your family? Do you spend time on your phone in bed when you could (or should) be winding your brain down to prepare it for sleep?

I was challenged about this very point by a delegate on one of my seminars who said that she always checked her phone before she went to sleep. By doing that, she knew there were no urgent messages from her children and that in itself relaxed her and helped her to get a good night's sleep. Who am I to argue with that? This is not an exact science, and in that case, it worked for her. Just something to consider for you and for those you support. First things first.

Police commanders were also culled in the financial crisis. On nights, it became usual for the night inspector to cover more than one division. This doubled your workload, literally overnight! Double staff, double the incidents to supervise, double the issues, double the threat, and sometimes higher than this, everything. In Greater Manchester, on nights, there is only one person working who is a higher rank to you. The Gold Commander. Generally, a superintendent, responsible for the more serious incidents. Murder, rape, serious car crashes, serious assaults, suspicious deaths, firearms incidents, anything to with terrorism and critical incidents. Anything which may have a significant impact on the community or threat to the reputation of the Force. The Gold

Commander's role was exceptionally busy, and they would not want to be mithered about anything to do with my workload!

When the pressure was on, it was common to have anything from 50 to 70 ongoing incidents to oversee. Some had rolled over from afternoons, and nothing would be happening with them overnight, although you still had to keep an eye on them in case there were overnight developments. There were always lots of missing people to find and a constant ebb and flow of incidents coming in and jobs being resulted by officers. All of this had to be overseen by me.

I pause here to send a huge shout out to the sergeants. Without them, my eyes and ears, I would be lost. They are, without doubt, the most important rank in the police service. They look after staff, manage incidents, document risk assessments, manage harm risk and threat for each incoming incident, missing person, or vulnerable person, allocate constables to incidents and attend serious incidents to take command and control. They are the gatekeepers who make sure nothing slips through the net. They are amazing human beings.

To help me manage everything, I used a simple technique. Everything I had responsibility for, all the incidents, missing people, welfare issues etc were recorded, each on one line of its own in my blue book. A lined hardback A4 journal.

Each was risk assessed and had a letter placed beside it.

M – Must do. The most urgent. The highest level of actual (or potential) risk of harm and threat to people or property.

S – Should do. Once the priority stuff is under control or completed. These were next.

C – Could do. Rarely done on nights because the more important stuff swallowed up all the resources I had. A careful watch was kept, though, in case anything changed with these overnight, raising the risk.

The benefits of this system are:

- It's easy to do.
- It helps you plan.
- It takes stuff out of your head to help you see things more clearly.
- It categorises your priorities and keeps first things first.
- It becomes a ready reference.
- You don't forget anything.
- It demonstrates your rationale/why you did things the way you did.
- It can be used during one-to-ones to decide priorities.
- It provides a record for you.

It's the power of three. This is my take on a traditional to-do list. Another thing you might like to try is having a 'to-not-do list'! We're particularly good at compiling lists of stuff we must do, but this is a way of decluttering your life. Start a list, at work or at home, in a diary. As you go about your day-to-day business, think about your routines and the things you do which don't serve any purpose or enrich your life. I came across this idea whilst reading an article from Harvard University in the United States and (like you might be now) was amused. I tried it and found it useful to reflect on my routines and tweak them to save time in my day. Even if you only come up with a handful of ideas and stop doing them (or tweak them), it's time saved for you. Give it a try!

Circles of influence

Who doesn't like a good moan? Putting the world to rights over a drink with friends or with neighbours over the garden fence has been a staple of British life for generations. Take the 'art' of queuing for example. The British are notoriously good at queuing whilst at the same time moaning about having to queue. We can moan when we're in a queue, moan about the length of the queue, moan about how slowly the queue's moving, moan about the person ahead of us holding up the queue. It's almost become a national pastime for some and has become fertile ground for scores of British comedians over the years. There's something cathartic about the moaning (huffing and puffing for those who are familiar with the term). *Get it off your chest. It's good to talk. A trouble shared is a trouble halved* were all things our grandparents used to tell us. And they were right.

Not for one second am I going to tell you that moaning, whinging, complaining (or whichever word you prefer) is bad for you. What I am advocating is balance and perspective with it. Specifically, being careful about how much time and energy you waste on things which you have no control over.

We have a term in the police for people like this. The 'mood hoover'. The person on the team who always had something to complain and whinge about. They attract other mood hoovers and generally have the same type of character so tend to stick together. Mood hoovers have the potential to affect the morale and wellbeing of a team in a negative way. Watch out for them, avoid them, and if you're the team leader, get a grip of them before they drag your team down.

Circles of influence is a simple way to restore balance and put time back in your 'time bank'. Equally as useable for you as it is as a coaching tool to help others. This is how it works.

Imagine a round target with three circular zones. The centre zone, the bullseye, is all about you and the choices you are free to make every day. What you eat, what you wear, the route you travel to work, what you'll do tonight, that kind of thing; it's all about you only. No issues with that, perfectly normal. The next ring, moving outwards, represents things you can have influence over. Choices at home and at work, the way you bring your children up, how you complete your work, how you spend your time, how you vote, who your friends are, the way you respond to situations, decision making and anything you have influence over. It's OK to spend time in this zone – it's productive. The final, outer ring represents things you have no control over whatsoever. This is the danger zone, the one which will steal your time, wear you down, exhaust your mental energy and generally not serve you well.

The point of this whole section is this. Be careful how much time and emotional energy you use up spending too much time in the outer circle. I'm not saying don't go there, that would be stupid, it's a perfectly natural and healthy place to be as long as you don't let it dominate your life. The football result for your favourite team last Saturday is important to you: it's outside your control and, therefore, in the outer zone, but it's important. Of course, you're going to talk, think, and expend energy thrashing out the detail of why the ref is useless, or the goalkeeper should be sacked! The point is, don't spend too much time there!

It's about recognising **when** you shouldn't be in the outer ring at all because it adds no value or positivity to your life at all.

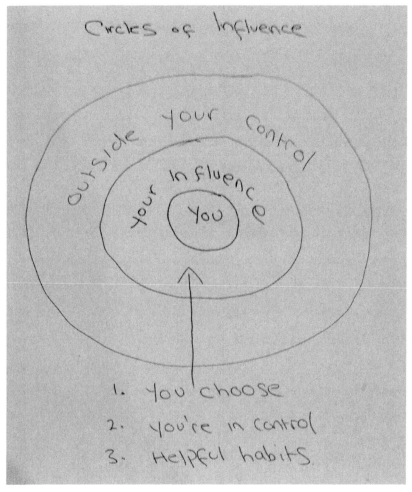

Circles of influence. Be careful of wasting time and emotional energy on things outside your control.

Promotion

A few years ago, Greater Manchester Police changed the promotion process for police sergeants going for promotion up to the rank of inspector. The chief constable, as you would imagine, took a keen interest in the process, wanting the best people for the job. No problem there.

The assessment process is competitive. It always has a paper application process, four interviews and role-play scenarios for candidates to showcase their skills, abilities, integrity, and ethics. This time it would be different.

In addition to the normal hurdles to overcome, the chief decided that every candidate had to record, and submit electronically a five-minute video of themselves, standing in front of their (imaginary) team and delivering a 'motivational briefing'. The video would be assessed by trained assessors with scores added into the overall assessment process. Well, this was completely different to anything the sergeants had been asked to do before and met with significant resistance. I can still recall the chatter in the offices, corridors, and canteens.

'He can't make us do this.' (Yes, he can; he's the chief, it's a lawful order and permitted under police regulations.)

'I'm not doing that.' (Don't do it then. Your choice. No video, no promotion.)

'It's a ridiculous idea.' (That's your opinion and you are entitled to it. Are you going to do it or not?)

The comments in brackets might sound harsh and a little abrupt but you can't argue with the facts. Let's not waste time here. All the negative comments, thoughts, and conversations about the fact that a video was needed sit firmly in the outer zone. Completely outside the sergeant's control.

What do you think the smart cookies were doing whilst all this was going on? Of course, directing their actions, thoughts, and energy, straight into the 'influence zone'.

'How do I do this?'

'Have I got the technical skill?'

'What do I need to research?'

'What kit do I need?'

'Do I need help from someone?'

'Where am I going to record it?'

'Should I be in uniform or plain clothes?'

'What will the content be?'

You get the idea?

In fact, the best story I heard was two sergeants who went to the media suite at Force Headquarters armed with chocolates, teabags, and biscuits and manged to persuade the staff there to let them record their videos in the video suite. A room normally reserved for press conferences, with smart logos, professional lighting and acoustics to match. Brilliant!

All positive stuff, rigidly fixed in the influence circle, which helped get their head in the right place and gave them the best chance of success.

Timing and a story about Fenty

Timing and knowing when, where, and how to use the tips, tools, and techniques in this book come from combining knowledge, practice, and experience, but not necessarily in that order.

Neil Fent or 'Fenty' as he was known, was what you would call an 'old school bobby'. Over six feet tall, wide at the shoulders and with an imposing presence. The sort of bobby your dad would reminisce about as being the one who would give you a 'clip round the ear' (followed by another off your mum and dad when you got home for getting caught in the first place!). Fenty had been a constable all his service and had twenty-five years 'in' when I first met him.

I liked him immediately. I could tell he had loads of experience as a 'copper'; he oozed confidence and made everyone, even newbies like me, feel welcome.

I knew from the start that working with Fenty would be good for me and jumped at the chance to be partnered with him at every opportunity. Not only did he know his stuff, but he also had a brilliant sense of humour and knew where to get the best 'Full English' on earlies.

Our callsign was November Mike Zero One. The subdivisional van working a 'two-ten' afternoon shift on a sunny Tuesday afternoon in May 1990.

The call was to a 'domestic'. Police language for some sort of family quarrel. Often minor in nature, but nothing taken for granted, as most murders committed in England are committed in family situations, often out of minor disagreements that boil up out of control.

We pull up outside the house, a terraced two-up two-down on a sprawling council estate. As we exit the van, the screaming and shouting from a male and female can be heard coming from the house, made easier by the front door being wide open.

Police officers have a lawful power of entry to go into an 'Englishman's castle', by force if needed, to protect life or prevent a breach of the peace. The racket coming from the house giving us a reason and lawful authority to enter. No force was needed that day; we walked straight into the hallway turning immediately right into the front room. Fenty went in first, I was just behind him.

We were met by Mr and Mrs Large standing nose to nose in the middle of the room and determined to carry on their slanging match, seemingly oblivious to the presence of the local constabulary in their living room.

I will never forget what happened next. It wasn't in the police manual of 'to deal with domestics' or written in any conflict management handbooks I know of, but it was incredible to see.

Fenty sat down on the settee and picked up a newspaper. Grabbing the remote control, he turned the television on and flicked to the horse racing pages on Ceefax (for younger readers, Ceefax is like Twitter on the telly but not as good!) The couple continued to rant as Fenty sat, cross-legged and relaxed, flicking his gaze between the paper and the telly. I stood in the doorway, dumbfounded, with no idea what was going on.

About fifteen seconds later, the couple slowly became aware that a policeman had walked into their living room and was sitting on the settee looking at the horse racing results on their telly!

They stopped rowing, both looking at Fenty with a look of horror and disbelief on their faces. Mr Large spoke first.

'What the fuck d'ya think you're doing!' he roared.

Fenty replied calmly and quietly with his gaze still fixed on the television.

'Hi folks, we've had a call about a disturbance from this house and I wondered if there was anything we can do to help, but before we do that, can I just check the 3.30 at York?'

I still had no idea what was going on, but what I did know was the fighting had stopped. Their attention diverted away from fighting each other and towards positive conversation to start resolving whatever the issue was. It was a surreal moment, but it worked!

Contrast that with a different approach, perhaps an attempt to verbally dominate the couple, put 'hands on' and start to wrestle them apart? Arrests, a fight, injuries, who knows? Gas, batons, handcuffs, Taser? Loads of options are available but communication skills, tact and diplomacy should always be the police officer's first choice.

Back to Fenty's technique. That was the first and last time I ever saw anyone, including Fenty, do anything like that. How did he know how to do that? How did he know he wouldn't make matters worse? Where on earth did it come from? He never disclosed.

'Experience, son!' was all I could ever coax from him.

The story was told many times at parties, retirement events; in fact, anytime we came together socially, invariably the story would be told, to peals of laughter.

No one can argue that it was unconventional, but it worked. It was exactly the right thing to do at that time. This story serves a purpose for us all. When we think about wellbeing, resilience and mental health, whether our own or someone else's, sometimes it takes something 'outside the box' to sort things out, and it often pays to be creative with what you do. There's no 'one size fits all', and timing is important, as it was for Fenty that day. Knowing what to do and when to do it will come to you too, as long as you remember that it all boils down to knowledge, experience, and practice, but not necessarily in that order.

Empathy

Empathy is the ability to sense other people's emotions coupled with the ability to imagine what they might be thinking or feeling. It is to put yourself metaphorically 'in their shoes' to try to understand and feel what they are going through. An important life skill, critical for good communication and essential for police officers.

Police officers need to be able to calm situations and communicate with people who are angry, stressed, emotionally charged and unpredictable. Empathy is the bedrock of good communication, and the best communication starts by trying to understand things from their perspective.

> Seek first to understand, then be understood.
>
> - Steven Covey *The 7 Habits of Highly Effective People*

You don't have to agree with someone to have empathy with them.

As a hostage and crisis negotiator, I don't agree with the man about to burn down the house he built for himself and his family just because his wife left him and took his children, but I do have empathy with him. The logic part of his brain has shut down. Why would he destroy all his hard work which cost him hours in blood, sweat, and toil, and thousands of pounds in materials? His emotional brain has taken over completely. He's hurt, angry, maybe jealous and his emotions are driving his behaviour. As soon as I recognise and understand this, I can start to respond in an empathic way to connect with him.

'You're not alone, I can help you and I'll stay as long as it takes to support you through this.'

'There is a way out of this for you, you have options, and it does not have to end badly for you.'

'I'm here for you, no matter what's happened we can work out a way through this together.'

'I've not experienced what you're going through, but I do understand your pain and I know you can get through this.'.

All supportive, all providing hope and providing choice and a way out for a man in crisis. Sometimes all people need is to be shown the way out.

The communication skills of hostage and crisis negotiators are outstanding. They listen with their ears, their eyes, and their hearts to understand. Looking and listening for 'hooks', tiny clues someone may divulge which the negotiator can use to influence things in a good way. The hook for this man was the love he had for his children and the love he'd ploughed into building a house for them. Both, understandably, very strong hooks to work with. The conversation led to this question and a turning point.

'Your kids love that you've built this house for them, and you know they will be back home at some point – do you think they'd miss playing in this house if it wasn't here?'

The man's thought patterns and perspective changed in an instant. From anger about his wife's actions, to not letting his children down, and the realisation, through floods of tears, about what he was about to do. His logical brain had kicked back in. The incident ended peacefully. No injuries and no requirement for the fire service, paramedics, or undertakers. There's a happy ending to this story. The man and his wife managed to resolve their differences and she moved back in with the children a week later. Empathy and understanding played their part in steering the conversation to help the man respond well, rather than react badly, and in making sure there was still a house for them all to move back into.

Empathy is a communication powerhouse and promotes understanding and connection with almost anyone. It reduces conflict and repairs damaged relationships quicker than almost anything else.

Monday 22 May will be forever in the memories of all those serving in Greater Manchester Police on that day.

The team response from Greater Manchester Police in the minutes, hours, days and weeks that followed was incredible. Whatever your role during that time, and as painful as the memories are, you should be proud of your contribution in supporting those affected and the city during the most challenging time in GMP history.

Ian Hopkins QPM
Chief Constable

The tiniest things often mean the most, don't they?

Muddy boots

I recall having a conversation with a sergeant called David during the wee small hours of a night shift. He told me he'd been having some arguments at home with his girlfriend, Amanda. David had been getting home from the night shift, about seven-thirty in the morning, tired and ready to go straight to bed. His muddy boots, which had seen plenty of overnight action, were kicked off and left in the kitchen by the back door. He was tired after a busy night and needed to get to sleep – his boots or, more specifically, where he'd left them of no major importance to him.

But it was to his girlfriend, Amanda! She loved him enough to have moved in with him recently and for the first few weeks everything was fine … until the boots … the muddy boots! Left for her to move (as she saw it) every morning and, even worse, 'left in the way for her to trip over and hurt herself.' She called him out on it and that's how the row started. It was important to her, but not to him and it went on, night after night, morning after morning, grinding them both down, yet neither 'giving in'. The more often he kicked his boots off and left them in the way, the more often she would (in his words) 'nag him'.

I listened to the story before replying.

'Why don't you just move your boots, David? Somebody's got to break the cycle, mate; why don't you be the bigger person and stop the quarrel?'

He looked indignant!

A fellow police officer! – a man! – taking sides with the 'enemy'!

Not at all!

It was never about taking sides (or gender). It was always about empathy and understanding the other person's perspective. An explanation of how empathy can resolve sealed the deal. I wanted Dave to try to understand things from Amanda's point of view and to show her that he understood the way she felt. I think he did. I think they're still happily together under one roof. Something tells me he moved his boots.

Advantages of empathy:

- It reduces conflict and helps to heal.
- It shows people you care and strengthens relationships.
- It allows you to become a better listener and, therefore, a better communicator.
- It allows you to become more receptive to new ideas and opportunities.
- It makes you a better leader and manager of people.
- It reduces everyone's stress levels and the need for you to tap into your resilience reserves.
- It's good for your mental health!

I highly recommend further study on the topic of empathy, and if this is new to you, here are three things to start you off on your journey to build more empathy into your life.

1. Learn to recognise emotions in other people and try to imagine what it feels like.

2. Develop your listening skills and the ability to ask sensitive questions with the sole intention of understanding more about what's going on for the other person.

3. Spend time with people who are different to you and practise one and two.

Forgiveness

Knowing which 'battles' to fight and how to forgive are important elements of building personal resilience. Do you get angry when someone 'does you wrong'? Do you hold grudges? Do you spend time plotting revenge or, worse still, get yourself into trouble because of it? Do you know people like this?

I've met police officers who've spent years waiting to get their own back on a colleague who didn't sign them off for promotion when they believed they deserved it, eaten up by a desire to 'pay them back' or obsessed about an ex-partner, deliberately sabotaging their life because they were jealous.

Experience shows that these things have a nasty habit of backfiring on you. And for those who believe that revenge is 'a dish best served cold', I suggest that outcomes rarely end well, especially when the police come knocking!

Forgiveness can be the hardest thing in the world. But it is possible. We see forgiveness from mothers whose children have been murdered – they say that forgiving the murderer helps them move on with their life. I cannot even begin to imagine how this works in practice, but I do know that forgiveness can be an incredible resilience-building tool (and spoke in your wheel), and if a bereaved mum can do it, maybe we can too. Forgiveness can neutralise anger and resentment, improve relationships and have a positive effect on physical health, improving mood, stress levels, blood pressure, and more.

I advocate 'forgiveness' to police officers knocking on my door wanting advice (or have been asked to come in for a chat) for all these reasons, and a conversation leading towards forgiveness can be navigated using the power of three and may go something like this:

Talk – Tell me what's bothering you. (Untangle the wool, dilute the acid, and make sense of what's happening.)

Soak time – Allow time for emotions to settle so they respond well rather than react badly to whatever the issue is. Ask questions and listen to understand.

Think – Enquire 'how important will this be in six months' time?' to help them gain perspective on what's important and make decisions which reflect the reality of the situation.

A simple three-step process like this will settle things down and can be used as many times as needed to help someone move on in a healthy, positive way.

Throughout this book, I've tried to ensure that you see the content as sharing useful tips, tools, and techniques with you rather than telling you what to do. It's the same here. All I ask is that you reflect on 'forgiveness' and where it sits with you, your character, and those around you. Most importantly, recognise whether forgiveness is in your armoury as a 'spoke', serving you well and supporting you positively. If it's not, then maybe this is your 'day one' to change things for the better. If it is, then please, pass it on and the next time someone approaches you and says, 'I cannot believe what so-and-so has just done to me!' you'll know immediately what to do!

Role models

I was an introverted, shy child, although those who know me as an adult may find this hard to believe! I've always had, what you might call, confidence issues, deep down. I wasn't academically bright; I was an immature boy (my teachers drummed this into me at every opportunity!) and always felt second best to everyone. I compensated for this lack of confidence and my poor social skills by reading. I loved reading. I had a thirst for knowledge and loved encyclopaedias more than anything. They were my window on the world. I was curious and had a thirst for knowledge. I wanted to learn how things worked, why things happened the way they did, and I was really interested in people, especially those who had achieved amazing things during their lives. I loved books about heroes too. Admiral Horatio Nelson was my favourite and a national icon. Britain's most famous naval commander, photographed by millions of tourists as a column topper in Trafalgar Square. You may know that Nelson died at the Battle of Trafalgar in 1805 just as he heard that his fleet had defeated the combined Spanish and French navies. An amazing piece of British naval history. Nelson was my first role model, but why and what's the connection with resilience?

During the 1700s, the Royal Navy was known for being a violent, unhealthy place to be. Dockyard towns were notorious for 'press-gangs' wandering the streets, skulking outside the many public houses where unsuspecting drunks were pounced on, often bludgeoned into unconsciousness, and forced to serve on warships. Men waking to greet their hangover on board a ship sailing out to sea. The ships themselves were inhumane, barbaric places where death and disease were never far away.

Nelson changed that. He was the first naval commander to care about his sailors. He made sure they were treated well and had more food than they could get on shore. They got fresh fruit, a daily allowance of grog (a mixture of rum and beer) and were paid well. It's reported that over three-quarters of the sailors who made up Nelson's Navy were volunteers rather than 'pressed men'. I remember reading this and being inspired. That was how I wanted to be known, as someone who cared about people. It seemed to me to be noble, right, and proper, and if it was good enough for Nelson, it was good enough for me! The seed was sown.

On the eve of the battle of Trafalgar, Nelson hoisted flags to communicate this famous line to the rest of his fleet.

England expects every man will do his duty.

His sailors were well prepared. Well fed, motivated, strong, and ready to go into battle. They were led by a brilliant warfare strategist who looked after his men. They would follow him anywhere. Those eight words sealed the victory, almost before a shot was fired. There was only going to be one winner.

Those words inspired me: 'England expects' and 'duty' became embedded in my DNA during my early life and throughout my career as a police officer. It meant something to me back then; it means something now.

We often think about role models as people we know now or have known, and that's true, but I also want to make the case that role models can also be our heroes and heroines from the past. I can, in an instant, dip into Nelson's story and use it to inspire me and push me on. It can be one of my 'three' at the drop of a hat if I choose it.

I encourage you to reflect on who your role models are. To think about why they inspire you and how you can embed that detail into your practice as one of your 'spokes'.

We also meet many role models throughout our lives. It can help to reflect and remember who they were and why they spring to mind as role models. What did they have that makes them stand out? How did they build resilience? Are these character traits you could adopt? By doing this as a reflective exercise, you may identify new spokes, tweaks to your own character or even identify the need for a complete overhaul.

This is what this exercise looks like for me.

Thank you. To the staff at Halfords in Blackpool in the 1980s for teaching me the value of honest hard work. To my driving instructor who taught me tolerance. To my tutor constable who taught me how to smile through difficult times. To the neighbourhood constable in Radcliffe who taught me empathy and compassion. To Barack Obama for demonstrating how to inspire with words and body language. To Steve Jobs who taught us to find work which made our 'heart sing'. To Mathew Syed for helping me 'reframe failure'. To Steven Covey for teaching me the seven habits of highly effective people. To the men and women of Greater Manchester Police who taught me how to carry on even though every nerve and fibre in my body said 'quit'. To Professor Steve Peters for introducing me to my 'chimp'. And to Jack, my friend aged 85 years who goes to my gym and gets up every time he falls.

Role models are everywhere, they are our spokes who help us build our resilience to incredible heights if we open our eyes, ears, and heart to let the learning in. Be open-minded, observant, curious, and consistent.

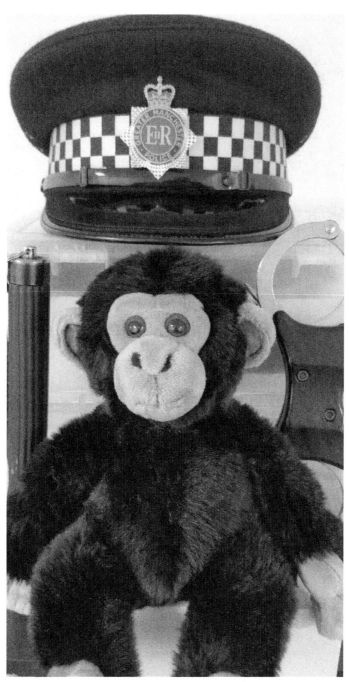

Millie plays a vital role during Safe and Sound training and always likes to be centre of attention!

You as a role model?

I'm going to keep this really brief because it is incredibly simple.

- If you develop a resilience practice and share what and how you do it, you will be an amazing role model.
- If you support others at every opportunity, you will be an amazing role model.
- If you go on to share the tips, tools, and techniques in this book, you will be a role model whose legacy will endure and be remembered forever.

What kind of role model do you want to be? ... Only you can answer that!

Sleep

Sleep deprivation has been used as a method of torture to 'grind people down' for centuries, and if you're one of the millions of people worldwide who don't get enough quality sleep, you'll get this!

It was the same in the police with shift work.

Your body clock (circadian rhythm, the experts call it) gets right out of sync when you're on earlies for a few days, then nights, then days off, then back on nights. Sometimes you don't know whether you're coming or going, and it will impact in some way:

performance at work, relationships at home, your happiness, and wellbeing.

Coming off a set of nights and into rest days was the worst for me. It could feel like being in some sort of twilight zone! You finish at seven o'clock in the morning, rush home and into bed for about eight o'clock with two choices…

One – force yourself out of bed about midday and spend the rest of the day feeling like a zombie in order to be tired enough to sleep that night.

Two – stay in bed all day and be wide awake watching the shopping channel on night-time TV a few hours later in the middle of the night.

Yes, working shifts can be tough on the mind and body. I feel much better nowadays now that I've had a 'normal' sleep pattern for a couple of years!

Poor quality sleep can grind you down, meaning lost mornings, bad moods and, potentially, poor health in the long term. I'm not a sleep expert by any means and don't claim to be. What I do share is the message that you don't have to suffer the effects of poor sleep, and even if this isn't an issue for you, it's worth learning more about it, having a greater understanding of why it's so important and having a few tips, tools, and techniques of your own to help others get a good night's sleep.

I overheard a sleep expert recently who shared his top tips for getting quality sleep.

- Open the bedroom windows slightly to circulate air around the room and maintain a cool temperature. Be warm under the duvet (but not too warm) but breathe cool air. This balance is scientifically proven to make it easier to get to sleep, and stay asleep, to get you into the deep sleep where proper rest and repair take place.

- Keep a journal at the side of your bed and record three good things which happened to you during the day. Doing this every night focuses your mind on something positive to think about as you drift off to sleep and will help you stay asleep. If you wake in the night with something on your mind, write it down. This empties your head and will help you get back to sleep.

- Don't have electronic devices in bed, as they stimulate the mind and waken it.

I was challenged about number three at a seminar I did. A lady came straight back at me to say that before she went to sleep, she always checked the messages on her phone to make sure none of her children needed her for anything. By doing that, she knew all was well and could go to sleep. I am not going to argue with that. It worked for her. It settled her down and helped her get good quality sleep. There are no hard and fast rules with stuff like this, often it's trial and error. What works for A won't work for B and vice versa.

I will always maintain that good quality sleep is essential to build unshakeable personal resilience and strong mental health for you and those around you. This singular topic is always worth reflecting on. For anyone wanting to learn more, there's loads more info available online at www.sleepcouncil.org

Choose your battles

Do you tend to get involved in everything that's going on and have an opinion on every topic? Do you constantly feel the need to take on every small argument at home or at work? Do you find yourself constantly at loggerheads with your partner, children, friends, or colleagues because of your need to be right? Are you stubborn and driven to win every time at any cost? (Sounds like the opening line to an advert doesn't it!)

If this is you or someone you know, I ask you to consider this:

'Is your need to fight every battle serving you well?'

There are many reasons why this can be a default response. Drive for perfection, lack of confidence, an ego or power thing, pride or habit ingrained since childhood. Experience shows that this habit can be damaging to your mental health because it wears you down. It's exhausting, affects the quality of relationships, steals your time, drains your energy, and erodes your resilience.

I met plenty of police officers like this. Often stressed, burned out or being disciplined because they'd 'snapped' and said or done something they shouldn't have because they just couldn't or wouldn't 'let it go'.

As a boss, I never tolerated bad behaviour by my officers. Period. I set the standard and led by example, a civil tongue and respectful behaviour. I expected my team to follow.

As well as setting the tone, it was my job to help police officers understand why fighting every battle was bad for them, and this is not just for police officers, this can affect us all if we let it.

An example from policing might be the new constable who's out on patrol for the first time on a Friday night at pub 'kicking out' time and hears the word PIG shouted at him by a drunk. Now the word pig is generally understood to be an insulting term to describe a police officer. The new officer, lacking in experience, immediately takes offence and approaches the man to exert his authority, thinking to himself, 'I'm a police officer now and the public are watching – nobody is going to embarrass or disrespect me!' The officer's ego has taken over, limiting their options to resolve calmly, and because of this, it's likely to end badly.

The officer marches over aggressively and with a stern voice and confrontational body language admonishes the male. The male takes offence at what he sees as an overbearing attitude by the officer, after all, he was 'only joking'. The officer raises his voice.

He feels like he's being made a fool of in front of everyone; his ego is bruised. He threatens to arrest the man if he dares to use 'abusive' language like that again. Within seconds, it's spiralling out of control. Both parties refuse to back down; members of the public are watching the scene unfold (people love to watch the police working as the number of reality TV shows demonstrates!).

Some of bystanders think the officer is being unreasonable – the man's apologised, the officer's making an issue out of nothing. They take the man's side and, all of a sudden, the officer is facing a group of ten annoyed drunks who are out to defend this man and the injustice of his treatment by the police. One against ten is never going to be good odds in a street fight. Thankfully, other officers intervene, and things settle down with no further problem.

This was a battle for that officer which did not need to be 'won'.

An off-the-cuff comment is never going to hurt anyone; in any case, it's not personal, it's directed at the uniform not me (how an experienced officer would view insults). It couldn't be directed at me personally: the drunk man doesn't even know me.

I'm going let the comment go. I'm going to make sure my body language and tone of voice are non-threatening and wander over to say hello. I'm going to be friendly and have a laugh and joke with him. Yes, that seems like a better option. He will feel a bit daft insulting a police officer who turned out to be a nice guy. The bystanders join in with a bit of banter, everyone smiling, laughing, and joking as they climb into taxis and go home. Job done.

The link to resilience is clear.

On the night, if the officer had got it wrong, he risked getting into a fight and getting injured. Maybe make an arrest. Would it be worth all the paperwork and time stuck in the station for one word? I think not. What if things had turned ugly? Could the officer have ended up being beaten up? Possibly, and for what, a one-word comment? Would that be worth it? Of course not. Would it affect the officer's confidence (and resilience) moving forward? Definitely.

It doesn't matter whether you're a police officer or not. I advocate choosing which battles to fight, and I'm hoping you're reflecting now. The insult example, or some other irritating issue, could happen at home or at work for you, with sons, daughters, partners, or colleagues. If you've been practising the tips, tools, and techniques I'm sharing, you will have plenty of spokes in place to respond well and not react badly and it won't be a problem, but if you consciously choose not to take on the battle in the first place, you won't need them!

These three questions are a guide to help you further.

- How important will this issue be in six months' time? If the answer is not important at all, why am I giving it any of my time and energy? Let it go.
- Is what I'm facing outside my control? If it is, there's nothing I can do about it. How much of my time, energy, and emotional energy am I going to waste getting involved?
- Would soak time' help things settle so I can make the best decisions moving forward?

The power of three as a personal mantra to help you but you must practice!

The serenity prayer

This prayer was displayed in my office at work. Wise words by a wise man and a brilliant example of the power of three.

God, grant me the serenity to accept the things I cannot change, courage to change the things I can and wisdom to know the difference.

- Reinhold Niebuhr (1892-1971)

Just get on with it!

As a resilience coach, I'm often confronted with the view that 'In my day, we just had to get on with it,' and I get that. I don't subscribe to it, but I get it. It's not my place to judge right or wrong and if 'just get on with it' keeps you going and works for you, that's great, however...

A word of caution and a question. If you adopt this mindset as your way of dealing with things, might you be storing up problems in the future for yourself by not offloading and decompressing?

Secondly, if your default position when advising and supporting someone else is to just get on with it, it probably isn't the right approach. In fact, it's highly likely to be the wrong approach.

Good examples to demonstrate this are ex-military personnel who gain huge benefits by talking about their experiences, in the right setting, with the right people. Talking is cathartic, an emotional release which can help lessen the impact and effects of post-traumatic stress disorder (PTSD).

On the battlefield, just getting on with it is what soldiers are trained to do (like policing on the front line, you have a job to do, you crack on and do it) but afterwards, when you leave the battlefield, it is good to talk, to offload, to decompress.

Resilience and leadership

There have been many books written about leadership. It isn't my intention to talk too much about the different types here, although it would be remiss of me not to talk about the role resilience plays for leaders and how your own personal resilience influences your behaviour as a leader. Quite often the term leader signifies the senior person, boss, manager, eldest, or group head. My definition is different. I want to make the case that anybody can be a leader and display leadership, particularly when it comes to wellbeing.

Demonstrating the tips, tools, and techniques in this book, by talking about them or using them to support others is leadership. It's not about job role, rank, or position in society. It is about care, compassion and stepping forward to help. On the night of the Manchester Arena attack, the city's taxi drivers stepped up. Despite the dangers, they gathered at the outer cordons, hundreds of them, desperate to help in any way they could. They transported the 'walking wounded' to hospital in their cabs, offered words of comfort to people shaking with fear and directed others to nearby hotels and other places of safety and refuge. They escorted ambulances through the chaos to reach the seriously injured and helped others navigate around the city. Just a few examples from one of many different groups who stepped forward that night. True leadership in action and something the people of Manchester will never forget.

Good leaders often make the best coaches and mentors when it comes to wellbeing because they care about their people. I define coaching as helping others achieve a specific personal or professional goal, and mentoring is an experienced person sharing what they know and how they do things to help train or guide a less experienced person. In this case, you, using your knowledge and experience for the benefit of others. There is a natural fit between leadership, coaching and mentoring and if you are in any leadership or management role, I encourage you to embrace all three to promote resilience, wellbeing, and strong mental health in your teams.

Leadership, coaching and mentoring combined. A bit of this, a bit of that, blurred edges but with a great result at the end of the day. No one size fits all. Every wellbeing situation and scenario unique.

Who were the best leaders during my thirty-year career?

Was it those who wore high-ranking epaulettes on the shoulders of their uniform and made the big decisions? Absolutely not. Some of the highest-ranking police officers were dreadful leaders. Many (including me) didn't trust them and wouldn't go to them unless we had to. We all knew who the trustworthy, honest, authentic leaders were.

Was it age? No. Some of the best leaders were the youngest on the team.

Was it because they were the best public speakers able to inspire the team? Partly. There is something about a leader's ability to inspire, motivate, and encourage by words, but that is not the be-all and end-all.

When I reflect on the question 'Who were the best leaders?' the answer I come to every time is this:

A good leader cares deeply about their team. They are authentic and honest in everything they do and can be trusted. They motivate, inspire, and empower everyone in the team to achieve amazing things. They know their job well but know their people better. They know what makes people tick and they demonstrate all these qualities, consistently, every single day.

The tips, tools, and techniques in this book will help you become an efficient, well-respected leader.

Be the change you want to see.
- Mahatma Gandhi

Bury BEE Well

June 2017

Supporting your welfare after the Manchester Arena attack

Inspector Russ Magnall

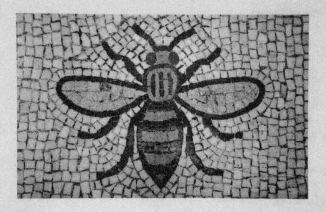

Over a short period of time, Manchester transformed at an astonishing rate from a small market town into a major industrial centre, processing 60% of the world's cotton. When Manchester was granted a coat of arms in 1842 its crest was adorned by seven bees placed upon a globe - the bees representing industry and the globe reflecting the city's global links.

Since then, the bee and the city have become symbolically interlinked. Businesses and events use the bee as a logo and design element to highlight their ties to Manchester. The Bee image above is from the mosaic floor at Manchester town hall. The symbol of the humble hardworking and resilient bee has also become a symbol of strength and unity in Manchester today.

Our greatest learning comes during our toughest times.

My top leadership tips

1. You must be authentic. It is no good 'talking the talk' if you don't 'walk the walk'. Combine what you already know with what you read in this book, and you will have an unbeatable combination. Consistency is key. People must see you living and breathing these tips, tools, and techniques.

2. You gain multiple benefits talking about resilience to large groups to promote your vision and set the tone for wellbeing culture, but that's not where trust is built. Trust is built during the hundreds and thousands of things you do and say, in the corridor, canteen, or at the water cooler to show you care.

3. 'My door is always open' must mean it! Put people first. Make sure your attitude, body language, tone of voice and response to the situation are genuine. Show that you mean it.

4. Whether it's a quick chat in the corridor or a more formal one-to-one where you provide support for someone, make sure you check back with them at some point in the future. How are things now? How is it going? You must consistently demonstrate your commitment to care.

5. Identify the 'influencers' in the team. People who 'get it' and will step up to proactively help others. Inspire and empower them into action. The Safe and Sound tips, tools, and

techniques are flexible. Share them with people around you and encourage them to get creative with them.

6. You must look after yourself. It isn't selfish to prioritise time to look after your own wellbeing. If you're not firing on all cylinders, you cannot look after those around you as well as you could. Too many people know this but don't do it! Don't be one of them.

7. I believe that sharing your story and bits about what's going on in your life is a good thing. Not the personal stuff talked about in a cringey way, but the stuff that shows you're human and have the same struggles, fears, worries, and concerns as them. Doing this displays honest authentic leadership and builds trust, and when you talk, it also gives your people permission to talk, which is a great thing. The term often used nowadays is 'psychological safety'. This is creating a culture where everyone feels free and safe to talk and express their thoughts and feelings in a way which won't be ridiculed or punished. They **feel** safe.

8. Leave this book where others will see it. Encourage people to talk about it. Invite challenge. Open as many conversations as you can about resilience, wellbeing, stress, and mental health.

Retirement

Why is this chapter at the end of the book when perhaps, it should have been at the start?

Is retirement (from the police service in this case) the end or the start? After all, retiring from the police has given me the opportunity, space, and time to write this. That's a start isn't it? The start of a new chapter if you excuse the pun!

And why is there a section about retirement in a book about resilience? Surely, you don't need any more resilience when you stop working, do you? I highlight stop working because I seem to have been busier since I left the police than I was when I was in it! Anyway I'm digressing. I'll get back to the point!

I'd attended the two-day pre-retirement course graciously provided by Greater Manchester Police in my final year of service. As a class, we were introduced to various wellbeing and financial experts to make sure we had all the advice we'd need to put all our 'ducks in a row' for a long and happy retirement.

I received loads of gifts and a cracking team photo on my last day as friends and colleagues bid me a fond farewell. I was asked, in front of about eighty people, to give a final speech. I cried. The emotion of the moment overwhelmed me. It had been a privilege to serve the communities of Greater Manchester for so long. I'd met thousands of amazing people over the years, laughed and cried with them and been involved in thousands and thousands of 'jobs'. All of this seemed to gang up on me and left me feeling very vulnerable standing there at the front of a crowded room as it dawned on me it was over. I walked out of the building with my head held high. My duty done.

My coaching work was picking up and I was getting busy catching up on all the stuff newly retired people do. Something was missing though. I missed the camaraderie, the banter, the social bit. It was the people. I missed the people … a lot.

If you've read the whole book, you'll be familiar with the well and wobble zones. I knew something wasn't quite right. Not quite a wobble, but I knew something wasn't quite right. I knew I needed to act and do something to correct matters. I connected with other retired police officers, in person and online. I talked about how I was feeling. I learned that this was normal and something most police officers feel when they retire. Sometimes it's immediate, sometimes it can take six to twelve months to kick in. I felt reassured. Talking had helped.

This strange and unfamiliar experience got me thinking. I'm a resilience coach, I know about stuff like this. I also had a plan for retirement, a strong support network around me, and on, I should have sailed through, but I found it a challenge. Thankfully, twelve months on, by talking, connecting with others, and leaning on my spokes, all was well.

I introduced retirement into my coaching programmes just as I left the police. I found it cathartic to talk to delegates about that bit of my journey. The here and now and where I was at that point in my life.

Many delegates open up about their own fears of impending retirement or share stories about partners retiring and the impact that's had on relationships and the dynamics in the house. Some of the stories are happy. Quite a few are not.

I talk about retirement in my Safe and Sound work today. My experience of retirement brings everything I share in this book about resilience right up to date and is as relevant for me now as it was when I started out all those years ago.

Be ready for it and remember, whatever you feel, it's normal and it will pass.

The journey continues. Keep well my friends.

Russ

Tips for coaches

1. There is no magic panacea when it comes to supporting the wellbeing of others, whether that's family and friends or in the workplace. Be creative. What works for one may not work for another, try things and practise. You won't go far wrong if you approach with a good dose of empathy and compassion.

2. Your leadership style is important. This is not about rank, role, or position in life. It's about your ability to step up when support is needed. Be open and honest to build trust and confidence in those around you. Be approachable, consistent, and authentic in everything you do. Build your character and great reputation will be yours for free.

3. Make wellbeing part of your daily practice. Demonstrate self-compassion and look after yourself. Doing this demonstrates the benefits to others and you subconsciously coach people because you are demonstrating good practice and leading by example. This makes you authentic and credible as a wellbeing coach.

4. Never overlook an opportunity to recruit more wellbeing champions. There will be people around you who have skills to support and it's incumbent on you to notice. Inspire and encourage willing talent to join your mission.

5. The simplest coaching models are the most effective. The GROW model:

- What are the **G**oals?
- What is the **R**eality?
- What **O**pportunities and **O**ptions are there?
- What is the **W**ork to do?

6. The power of **three Cs** works 'in the moment':

- **C**onfirm: (what's going on here?)
- **C**onsider: (What three things will I use now?)
- **C**ontinue: (Move forward, no matter how slowly)

7. Be mindful of your communication style. What you say and how you say it. Be mindful of your body language. Is it congruent with your message and what you are trying to achieve? (The bestselling book **Verbal Judo** by Dr George Thompson is an excellent resource for coaches wishing to improve their communication ability and is in my top three all-time best books.)

8. Do not be afraid to talk about how you are – when you talk, you give others permission to talk too. Talking is a good thing, especially about emotions, thoughts, feelings, mental health, and wellbeing. By getting people talking about wellbeing, we change wellbeing culture for the better.

9. The number one communication skill is listening. Practise every day. Your goal is to listen to understand. Be wary of falling into the trap of appearing to listen but, actually, just waiting for your turn to reply.

Seek first to understand, then to be understood.

- Steven Covey The 7 Habits of Highly Effective People

10. Stay curious and ask open questions which don't invite a yes or response. (Why? What? Who? When? Where?) Open, constructive questions generate much better-quality conversations.

11. Don't be afraid of silence when having wellbeing conversations. One of the traps for coaches is feeling awkward about silence. If the person you're with isn't talking, you may feel the need to fill the gap. Silence is an incredible wellbeing tool in its own right because it allows people space and time to think and rationalise their thoughts (soak time). If this approach doesn't come naturally to you, it's worth practising with people around you under 'normal conditions' so that you become more comfortable with the technique as a wellbeing coach.

12. Seemingly small things to you are big things to others. Sweat the small stuff.

13. Don't let the small things carry on growing into big things. If you are blessed with a managerial or leadership position, you must have the courage to nip things in the bud and have difficult conversations when needed. Things which cause upset and fester in the workplace will have a direct impact on the wellbeing of staff and the team as a whole. Examples might be gossiping, a misplaced sexist or insulting comment or acquiescing to unacceptable workplace culture. Familiarise yourself with the term 'microaggressions' and build prevention into your practice.

14. Don't shy away from conversations which encourage others to take responsibility for their own wellbeing. We all have a responsibility, and it is not **solely** the responsibility of you, the team, the company, or the individual's family to look after them. This can be a tough message to hear for some, so needs to be approached at the right time and with care and sensitivity. We are all in this together and we all have a role to play to keep ourselves fit and well.

15. Commit to a life of constant and consistent growth and most of all … PRACTISE!

As long as you've got air and can breathe
everything else can be worked out.

- Greater Manchester Police Underwater
Search Team Survival Training

Contact Russ about his Safe & Sound workshops on LinkedIn or
russellmagnall@gmail.com

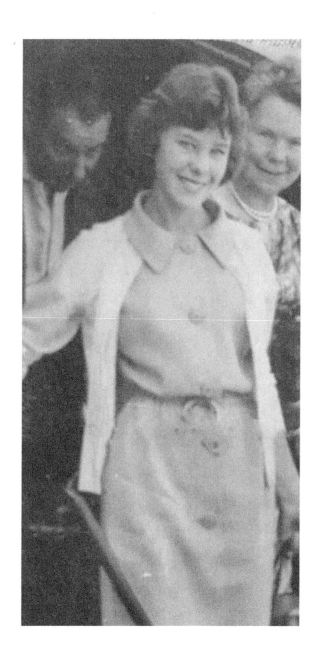

My mum. "Be careful crossing the road Russell, I want you back Safe and Sound." Hope I did you proud, Mum.

Printed in Great Britain
by Amazon